D0416827

**PUBLISHERS NOTICE**

As of August 1994, readers are
advised that the prescribing status
of felbamate in the United States of
America and all other markets
where it is available is currently
under review following reports of
aplastic anaemia

# New Anticonvulsants
Advances in the Treatment of Epilepsy

# New Anticonvulsants
## Advances in the Treatment of Epilepsy

*Edited by*

M.R. TRIMBLE

*Department of Neurology,*
*Institute of Neurology,*
*Queen Square,*
*London,*
*UK*

JOHN WILEY & SONS
Chichester · New York · Brisbane · Toronto · Singapore

*Other Wiley Editorial Offices*

John Wiley & Sons, Inc., 605 Third Avenue,
New York, NY 10158–0012, USA

Jacaranda Wiley Ltd, 33 Park Road, Milton,
Queensland 4064, Australia

John Wiley & Sons (Canada) Ltd, 22 Worcester Road,
Rexdale, Ontario M9W 1L1, Canada

John Wiley & Sons (SEA) Pte Ltd, 37 Jalan Pemimpin #05-04,
Block B, Union Industrial Building, Singapore 2057

*Library of Congress Cataloging-in-Publication Data*

New anticonvulsants: advances in the treatment of epilepsy
    edited by M. R. Trimble.
        p.   cm.
    Includes bibliographical references and index.
    ISBN 0 471 95122 6
    1. Anticonvulsants.   I. Trimble, Michael R.
    [DNLM: 1. Anticonvulsants—pharmacology.   2. Anticonvulsants—
therapeutic use.   3. Epilepsy—drug therapy.   QV 85 N 53165 1994]
    RM322.N47   1994
    615′.784—dc20
    DNLM/DLC
    for Library of Congress                                    94-9621
                                                                  CIP

*British Library Cataloguing in Publication Data*

A catalogue record for this book is available from the British Library

ISBN 0 471 95122 6

Typeset in 10/12pt Times by Dorwyn Ltd, Rowlands Castle, Hants
Printed and bound in Great Britain by
Biddles Ltd, Guildford and King's Lynn

# Contents

# Contributors

Martin J. Brodie, *Epilepsy Research Unit, Department of Medicine and Therapeutics, Western Infirmary, Glasgow, G11 6NT, UK*

David Chadwick, *Walton Centre for Neurology and Neurosurgery, Rice Lane, Liverpool, L9 1AE, UK*

W. Edwin Dodson, *St Louis Children's Hospital, One Children's Place, St Louis, Missouri 63110, USA*

John S. Duncan, *Institute of Neurology, Queen Square, London WC1N 3BG, UK*

Lennart Gram, *University Clinic of Neurology, Hvidovre Hospital, DK-2650 Hvidovre, Denmark*

Kevin M. Kelly, *Department of Neurology, University of Michigan Medical Center, Ann Arbor, Michigan 48104-1687, USA*

Ilo E. Leppik, *Department of Neurology, University of Minnesota, 5775 Wayzata Blvd, Minneapolis, Minnesota 55416-1222, USA*

Robert L. Macdonald, *University of Michigan Medical School, Neuroscience Laboratory Building, 1103 East Huron Street, Ann Arbor, Michigan 48104-1687, USA*

Paul J.W. McKee, *Epilepsy Research Unit, Department of Medicine and Therapeutics, Western Infirmary, Glasgow G11 6NT, UK*

John M. Pellock, *Department of Neurology, Randolph Manor Hall, Medical College of Virginia, 307 College Street, Richmond, Virginia 23298, USA*

Emilio Perucca, *Clinical Pharmacology Unit, Piazza Botta 10, 27100 Pavia, Italy*

Anne Sabers, *University Clinic of Neurology, Hvidovre Hospital, DK-2650 Hvidovre, Denmark*

Michael R. Trimble, *Institute of Neurology, Queen Square, London WC1N 3BG, UK*

# Preface

The management of epilepsy is no longer a simple process. Gone are the days when there were only a couple of useful drugs, no serum level monitoring, and uninformed patients. The last 20 years have seen the introduction of many significant advances for the care of patients with epilepsy. Notable are the use of plasma level measurements to obtain, with some drugs, appropriate therapeutic levels or the avoidance of toxicity; the better definition of seizure types to be treated, by such techniques as video telemetry and the application of internationally recognized classifications of seizures and underlying syndromes; and the use of surgery for well-designated patients following intensive monitoring.

Of utmost significance has been the introduction of new anticonvulsant drugs. The 'second generation' compounds, until recently referred to as new, such as carbamazepine and valproate, have been used world-wide. Their therapeutic profile is largely known, their toxicity understood, and all physicians looking after patients with epilepsy have extensive experience with them. It is usually acknowledged that some 60–80% of new-onset patients achieve excellent seizure control with these drugs — a remarkable achievement. However, in a significant proportion of patients attacks continue relentlessly, which ultimately takes its toll of the patients' psychosocial, and often physical, well-being.

The pharmaceutical industry has not been idle in attempting to ameliorate the plight of this group of patients, and some of the neuroscience innovations of the 1980s have delivered for the 1990s a collection of new anticonvulsant drugs. Indeed, they are a collection, each probably with differing modes of action and spectra of clinical activity.

Thus, the medical management of epilepsy has become very complicated. There is now a plethora of drugs to use, meaning greater opportunities for effective seizure control, but also more interactions, differing side-effect profiles, and, perhaps most worryingly, the potential for a return to unbridled, irrational polypharmacy.

It is in this light that this book was conceived. It was recognized by the editor that there is some, often inadequate, educational material about these drugs available. However, much of this is generated by the pharmaceutical industry itself, potentially biasing the information available, for example concentrating the text largely on one drug to the exclusion of the rest. There are some large texts available where some of the information contained in this book can be found. However, at present, there are few sources for the interested reader of up-to-date clinical information on the new drugs. This book is intended to fill the gap, for a time at least.

It has to be recognized that our information about the new drugs is inadequate in many areas, and for some drugs even the most experienced investigators have limited experience. However, it is hoped that the book will be a useful clinical text for those wishing to update their knowledge in this important therapeutic area.

The book is strictly limited in its scope. It does not cover the numerous drugs in development that may become available in future years, and is concerned only with those clinically available in some countries at the present time. It is envisaged that the drugs to which an entire chapter is devoted will be widely available in the near future.

There may be some who feel that other drugs should have been included, but this would have taken away the emphasis on current clinical practice. To my knowledge, zonisamide is perhaps the main omission, but it is not available as yet anywhere in the Western world, and its future status remains uncertain. It is discussed briefly in Chapter 10.

The first chapter is an overview of pharmacokinetics. This was intended to refresh the reader's knowledge of some fundamental principles, and then apply them to the new drugs. This is followed by discussion of potential mechanisms of action, before the chapters devoted to individual drugs. The latter cover clobazam, an old drug in some countries, but a new one in others, gabapentin, felbamate, lamotrigine, oxcarbazepine and vigabatrin. The current position on prescribing for children is then presented, before the final chapter which summarizes the current role of the new drugs from the point of view of one experienced clinician investigator, a difficult task at the best of times, but particularly difficult in our present state of knowledge. The opinions stated are entirely those of the author.

In editing these contributions I have tried to draw a balance between repetition of facts about individual drugs, and keeping each chapter as readable and complete as possible.

The opinions presented are entirely those of the individual authors, to whom I am grateful for their time and effort in producing their manuscripts. It is hoped that this book will prove useful to those clinicians, and others involved in the management of epilepsy, who require an up-to-date summary of new anticonvulsant drugs.

M.R.T.
*London, January 1994*

# Conversion factors for drug concentration measurements

To convert µg/ml to µmol/l multiply drug concentration by the factors indicated.

| ANTIEPILEPTIC DRUG | CONVERSION FACTOR |
|---|---|
| Carbamazepine | 4.23 |
| Carbamazepine-Epoxide | 3.96 |
| Clobazam | 3.33 |
| Clonazepam | 3.17 |
| Gabapentin | 5.83 |
| Lamotrigine | 3.90 |
| *N*-Desmethyl Clobazam | 3.49 |
| Oxcarbazepine (OXC) | 3.96 |
| OXC metabolite (10-OH) | 3.96 |
| Phenobarbitone | 4.31 |
| Phenytoin | 3.96 |
| Primidone | 4.58 |
| Valproic Acid | 6.93 |
| Vigabatrin | 7.74 |

# 1

# Pharmacokinetic interactions with anticonvulsant drugs

PAUL J. W. MCKEE AND MARTIN J. BRODIE
*Western Infirmary, Glasgow, UK*

## INTRODUCTION

Complete control of epileptic seizures using a single anticonvulsant drug can be anticipated in fewer than 80% of patients (Brodie, 1990). The remainder will receive polypharmacy despite little evidence of substantial improvement in the majority. In addition, combinations of anticonvulsant drugs often result in complex and unpredictable interactions. The greater the number of drugs the patients take, the more likely they are to experience an adverse reaction (Petrie and Cluff, 1980). Fortunately, only a small proportion of potential interactions have clinical repercussions. Knowing the pharmacology of the drugs, appreciating the likely underlying mechanisms and identifying the most vulnerable patients will anticipate many adverse interactions and promote safer prescribing.

## HIGH-RISK DRUGS

High-risk drugs are agents in widespread clinical use with marked efficacy and a narrow therapeutic index. Small changes in circulating concentrations may result in loss of clinical effect or precipitate toxicity. Phenytoin is particularly susceptible to inhibitory interactions as it undergoes saturable hepatic metabolism. With carbamazepine, autoinduction of metabolism produces a pure population of enzymes that provide a prime target for inhibitors.

*New Anticonvulsants: Advances in the Treatment of Epilepsy.* Edited by M. R. Trimble
© 1994 John Wiley & Sons Ltd

## VULNERABLE PATIENTS

Patients at greatest risk of experiencing deleterious adverse effects as a consequence of a drug interaction are the elderly, the severely ill and those individuals taking several drugs concurrently (Brodie and Feely, 1988). Patients with refractory epilepsy fall particularly into this last category. In addition, a breakthrough seizure may be a disaster for a patient with previously well-controlled epilepsy who perhaps drives; an unwanted pregnancy in a young woman relying on oral contraception would be similarly disastrous.

## PHARMACOLOGICAL THEORY

Conventionally, a drug interaction can be regarded as the modification of the effect of one drug by prior or concomitant administration of another. A more correct definition might insist that the pharmacological outcome of such a combination be more than just an additive function of their individual effects. The resultant response must be greater (potentiate) or less (antagonize) than the sum of their separate actions (McInnes and Brodie, 1988).

Adverse drug interactions can be conveniently divided into those involving the pharmacokinetics of a drug and those influencing the pharmacodynamic response to it. Pharmacokinetic interactions can affect absorption, distribution, metabolism or excretion. Owing to marked interindividual variability in these events, they can be anticipated, but their extent cannot readily be predicted. Pharmacodynamic interactions are less easily classifiable. They may be inferred from the production of synergism or antagonism to the beneficial or adverse effects of two drugs without change in concentration of either (McInnes and Brodie, 1988). This chapter concentrates on pharmacokinetic interactions.

## GLOSSARY OF PHARMACOLOGICAL TERMS

### Absorption

Although absorption takes place throughout the gastrointestinal tract, the major site is in the upper small bowel, whose surface area is equivalent to two full-sized tennis courts. Lipid-soluble drugs are rapidly absorbed by passive diffusion. Absorption of water-soluble compounds is slower and may be incomplete. The time to peak plasma concentration is usually around 1–3 hours after ingestion unless gastric emptying is slowed, which can occur physiologically following a heavy meal, pathologically during severe pain, and pharmacologically due to opiates, tricyclic antidepressants and neuroleptics. This results in a delayed and attenuated peak drug concentration and effect. However, the amount of drug absorbed is not usually reduced as compensatory absorption occurs further down the gastrointestinal tract. Extensive small bowel pathology has little effect on the bioavailability of lipid-soluble drugs. The absorption of a water-soluble drug is more likely to be incomplete.

## Accumulation

Accumulation occurs when repeated dosing with a drug leads to a gradually increasing amount in the body. It is a particular problem with agents that undergo saturable hepatic metabolism (such as phenytoin) or substantial first-pass metabolism (such as verapamil). Accumulation occurs to a lesser extent with drugs that have an elimination half-life exceeding 24 hours. As drug elimination is slower in the elderly, accumulation occurs more often in this patient population.

## Bioavailability

Bioavailability is the term used to describe the percentage of an oral dose reaching the systemic circulation and hence the site of action. It depends on the extent of absorption (usually nearly complete) and, more importantly, the amount of drug metabolized on the 'first pass' through the gut wall and liver. As drug injected intravenously can be regarded as 100% bioavailable, oral bioavailability can be calculated as the ratio of the areas under the oral and intravenous concentration–time curves following a single dose given by both routes (Figure 1).

## Clearance

The clearance of a drug can be obtained from the dose administered divided by the area under concentration–time curve. It is usually expressed as volume of plasma cleared of drug per unit time. Total clearance is often a composite of renal and hepatic clearances and is independent of the volume of distribution.

## Distribution

The distribution of a drug can be regarded as its reversible transfer throughout the vascular compartment, extracellular fluid and tissues. The volume of distribution is a convenient mathematical term that assumes that the drug is present throughout the body in the same concentration as in the plasma. It is calculated by dividing an intravenous dose by the estimated drug

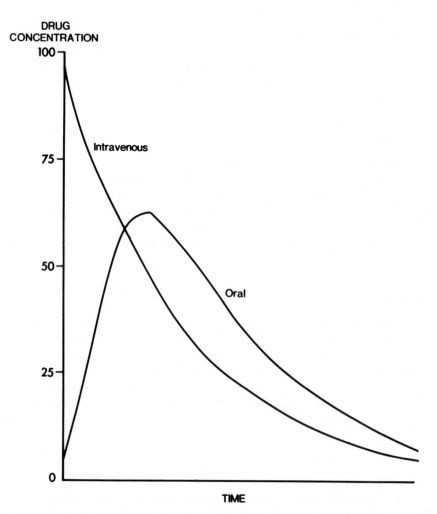

**Figure 1.**   Superimposed concentration–time curves for the same dose of a drug given intravenously and orally. The bioavailability is calculated as a ratio of the area under the oral curve as a percentage of the intravenous. In this case bioavailability approximates to 100%

concentration at the time of injection ($C_0$); $C_0$ can be obtained by extrapolating to time zero from the log-linear concentration–time curve (Figure 2). Volume is usually expressed in litres and provides a measure of the amount of a drug load remaining in plasma and that present in tissues. Thus, if all the drug were confined to the vascular compartment, the volume of distribution would be around 5 litres. Volumes over 250 litres suggest most of the drug is bound in the tissues.

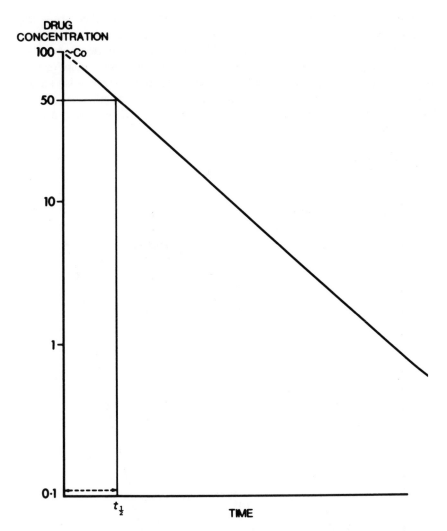

**Figure 2.** Concentration–time curve for a drug given intravenously with the concentration plotted on a logarithmic scale. The estimated plasma concentration at the time of injection $(C_0)$ can be obtained by extrapolating the line backwards to the vertical axis—in this case 100 units. Volume of distribution can then be calculated as dose/$C_0$. The elimination half-life $(t_{1/2})$ can be read off as the time taken for the concentration of the drug to fall by half, e.g. from 100 to 50 units

## Dose response

The pharmacodynamic response to a drug can be related to its concentration at the site of action and, therefore, the dose administered. There is a minimum dose at which an effect is detectable and a higher one where maximal change is produced above which no further increase is possible. By plotting the dose on a logarithmic scale, the typical S-shaped curve can be obtained (Figure 3). Generally, drugs exhibiting a flat dose–response curve are easier to use clinically than those with a steep dose–response curve, as fewer dosage increments are needed to obtain a satisfactory response. Dose–response relationships for concentration-related toxicity run parallel to the efficacy curves.

**RESPONSE**

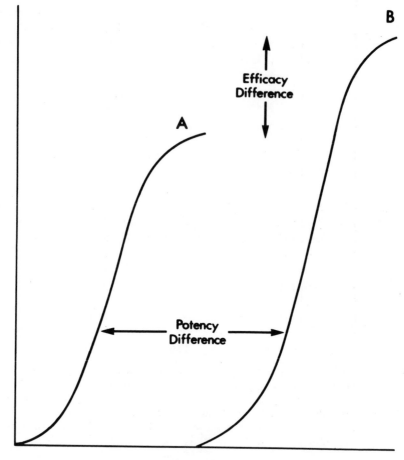

**Log Drug Dose**

**Figure 3.**   Log dose–response curves for drugs A and B. Drug A (e.g. bendrofluazide) is more potent than B, but B (e.g. frusemide) is more effective than A (as a diuretic but not as an antihypertensive!)

## Elimination

Drug elimination represents its irreversible loss from the body, largely by metabolism in the liver, excretion by the kidneys or a combination of both. Metabolites can be excreted in the bile and urine.

## First-pass metabolism

A number of drugs, when given orally, undergo substantial metabolism on the first pass through the gut wall, liver or both. As a result less than 30% of a single dose will reach the systemic circulation and its site of action. As this metabolism is saturable, a 40-fold variation in peak plasma concentration may be anticipated following the same oral dose given to a number of patients. On chronic dosing, steady state levels are higher than expected and may vary five-fold. In patients with hepatic cirrhosis, bypassing of hepatic metabolism by portosystemic shunting will markedly augment oral bioavailability. Enzyme inducers decrease and enzyme inhibitors increase the bioavailability of drugs with a high first-pass metabolism.

## Half-life

The elimination half-life of a drug represents the time taken for its concentration in the plasma to fall by 50%. When a drug is given intravenously and blood is removed frequently over a sufficiently long period, a concentration–time curve can be constructed (see Figure 2). For most drugs the amount eliminated from the plasma is directly proportional to the amount present, i.e. first-order kinetics prevail. Plotting the concentration on a logarithmic scale transforms the curve into a straight line. The half-life of the drug can then be easily read. The concentration–time curve following an oral dose is more complicated as the drug must be absorbed and distributed before undergoing elimination. However, when the concentration is plotted on a logarithmic scale, the declining part of the curve will usually be a straight line and the elimination half-life again readily obtained.

## Metabolism

Lipid-soluble substances must be transformed to water-soluble products prior to efficient elimination from the body. The liver is the major metabolic factory. Many drugs undergo two phases of metabolism, namely oxidation and conjugation (Figure 4). The phase 1 enzymes responsible for oxidation and similar reactions are known as mono-oxygenases, and can be collectively measured in liver tissue as cytochrome P450. The metabolites produced are usually inert. Although some do have biological activity, this is usually less

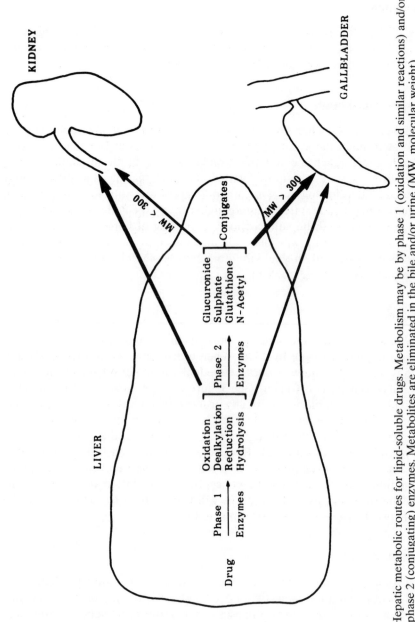

**Figure 4.** Hepatic metabolic routes for lipid-soluble drugs. Metabolism may be by phase 1 (oxidation and similar reactions) and/or phase 2 (conjugating) enzymes. Metabolites are eliminated in the bile and/or urine (MW, molecular weight)

than with the parent compound. Rarely, a toxic substance (e.g. paracetamol) or even a carcinogen (e.g. benzypyrene) can be formed. Some pro-drugs, such as oxcarbazepine, have to be metabolized in the liver to provide the active moiety. Products of oxidative reactions are eliminated directly in urine or bile or further metabolized by conjugation via phase 2 enzymes. Conjugation involves the addition of an endogenous substance, such as sulphate or glucuronic acid, to produce a more polar molecule. Some drugs are metabolized only by conjugation. Almost all conjugates are inert. Larger drugs and metabolites are excreted in bile whereas smaller ones (molecular weight less than 300) pass out in the urine.

Premature infants have impaired drug metabolism, whereas young children often eliminate lipid-soluble drugs more rapidly than do adults. Thereafter, the activity of these enzymes gradually tails off into old age. Patients with cirrhosis should be prescribed initially half the standard dose of a drug primarily eliminated by oxidative processes. Conjugated drugs can be given in standard doses until clinical signs of hepatic decompensation supervene.

For most drugs in clinical use, first-order kinetics apply, i.e. the rate of elimination from the body is directly proportional to the circulating concentration. For a few agents (e.g. phenytoin) the liver's capacity to remove the drug can be saturated and further drug metabolism is subject to zero-order kinetics. Under these conditions, a modest increment in phenytoin dose, for instance, can result in substantial increase in concentration with resultant neurotoxicity (Figure 5). Conversely, a modest reduction in dose may produce an unexpectedly substantial fall in phenytoin level, resulting perhaps in seizure breakthrough.

### Potency and efficacy

The potency of a drug is defined by its position along the horizontal axis of its dose–response curve (see Figure 3). The more potent the drug, the lower the dose required to produce a pharmacological response. The efficacy of a drug is the extent of the response it produces. Potency differences can be overcome by giving the patient a higher dose, but maximal efficacy cannot be improved upon. In clinical practice potency has little relevance. When you see the term 'potency' in a review, the authors probably meant 'efficacy'!

### Protein binding

Some acidic and neutral drugs bind to serum albumin, while basic drugs bind to globulins and acute phase reactants, such as alpha-1 acid glycoprotein. Protein binding is rarely of clinical relevance and only theoretically relevant for drugs more than 90% bound to plasma proteins. In chronic dosing, unbound (free) drug is responsible for its pharmacological and toxic effects

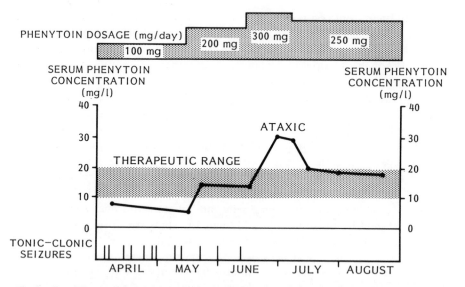

**Figure 5.** Effect of increasing phenytoin dosage on seizure frequency and serum phenytoin concentration in a 75-year-old man with secondary generalized tonic–clonic seizures following a cerebrovascular accident. On increasing the phenytoin dosage from 200 mg to 300 mg daily, the plasma concentration trebled and signs of ataxia were apparent. On reducing the dose by only 50 mg, the phenytoin concentration re-entered the target range and seizure control was maintained without side-effects

(Figure 6). If protein binding is reduced by disease or by competition with another drug, more unbound drug is available for metabolism and a similar free concentration is attained to that circulating prior to the alteration in binding. However, a compensatory fall in total drug concentration occurs. This may stimulate an unnecessary change in drug dosage by the doctor, who is mesmerized by a measured drug concentration. In disease states that result in lowered albumin levels (e.g. nephrotic syndrome) binding of phenytoin may be reduced, whereas increased binding of carbamazepine may occur following myocardial infarction (McInnes and Brodie, 1988).

### Renal excretion

After glomerular filtration, lipid-soluble drugs and metabolites diffuse back passively into tubular cells and re-enter the circulation, whereas water-soluble drugs and metabolites are eliminated in the urine. The renal tubular system also actively secretes drugs. There are specific mechanisms for the secretion of acidic and basic substances for which some drugs compete (McInnes and Brodie, 1988).

A few substances depend on renal excretion alone for elimination without prior oxidation or conjugation in the liver. For these water-soluble molecules,

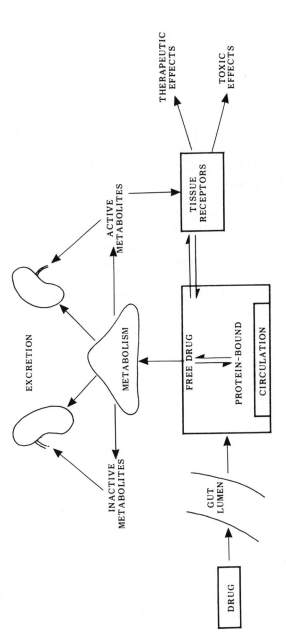

**Figure 6.** Relationship between bound and free drug. Bound drug is trapped in the vascular space, whereas unbound (free) drug is distributed throughout the tissues and is responsible for its pharmacological and toxic effects. The higher the amount unbound, the greater its availability for hepatic metabolism or renal excretion

clearance is dependent on glomerular filtration rate. If the drug has a narrow therapeutic ratio, dosage must be adjusted in relation to impairment of renal function, which can be most conveniently measured using the serum creatinine.

## Steady state

When a number of doses are given over a period of time, eventually the amount of drug absorbed is similar to that eliminated from the body, i.e. equilibrium or steady state has been reached. The time taken for a drug to attain steady state is a mathematical function of its elimination half-life. Thus, after one half-life 50% of steady state is achieved, 75% after two, 87.5% after three and so on. For practical purposes, steady state can be anticipated after five half-lives (Figure 7). Knowledge of the half-life of a drug can be useful, if the concentration is closely related to its pharmacological effect. For such agents it allows prediction of the approximate time to maximum effect both on initiating therapy and changing the dose. Similarly the rate of decay in response can be anticipated when the drug is discontinued.

The steady state concentration of a drug represents the average value throughout the day. In reality the concentration varies constantly as new drug

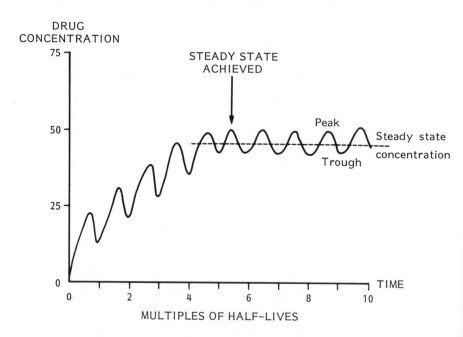

**Figure 7.** Concentration–time curve on initiating chronic drug therapy. Steady state is reached after about five elimination half-lives

is absorbed and that circulating is metabolized and excreted. This results in a number of peaks and troughs. Their magnitude depends on the elimination half-life and the frequency of dosing (Figure 7). Thus, for some drugs with a half-life exceeding 24 hours, such as phenobarbitone, a single daily dose will provide acceptable steady state concentrations. However, such an approach may also produce a high peak concentration several hours after dosing, which may cause unacceptable sedation. Dividing the dose may improve tolerability, but at the expense of compliance. For most drugs high peaks and low troughs are best avoided, and a true steady state with no hour-to-hour variation would be ideal. This can be attained only with an intravenous infusion. Modified-release versions of certain drugs have been developed, e.g. carbamazepine and sodium valproate, in an attempt to reduce the diurnal fluctuations in serum levels found with the established formulations.

## THERAPEUTIC DRUG MONITORING

Measurement of the serum drug concentration was developed to help explain some of the observed variation in individual response to drug action. From these early beginnings the 'science' of therapeutic drug monitoring has evolved to include manipulation of the drug dosage to bring the concentration within a predetermined range (Spector *et al.*, 1988). Implicit in its appropriate clinical use is the requirement that the concentration correlates better with clinical effect and toxicity than the dose. Although not part of the purist's definition, many physicians have extended its practical application to checking compliance.

The pharmacological characteristics of some of the established anticonvulsant drugs make them suitable candidates for therapeutic drug monitoring. Phenytoin best fulfils the criteria, as its saturable kinetics make it difficult to choose the correct dose without measuring the circulating concentration (Brodie, 1990). Because of the presence of active metabolites and the marked variation in concentrations during a dosage interval, there is a poor correlation between circulating levels of carbamazepine and sodium valproate, and anticonvulsant effect and central nervous system toxicity (Brodie and Feely, 1988). The value of measuring phenobarbitone is also limited, as concentrations associated with optimal control vary considerably; in addition, the development of tolerance to its central nervous system side-effects makes the toxic threshold imprecise. With ethosuximide, the clinical status of the patient and the presence or otherwise of gastrointestinal or central nervous system side-effects can usually be readily assessed without recourse to concentration measurement.

Although monitoring anticonvulsant levels can be helpful in optimizing the dosage in some patients, rigorous adherence to a particular range is likely to result in the doctor treating the drug concentration and not the patient

(Larkin *et al.*, 1991a). The 'therapeutic' or, better, 'target' range can only be regarded as an approximation, based as it is on population data. Some patients will do well with levels below the lower limit of the target, whereas others will tolerate concentrations well above the range with benefit (Brodie and Feely, 1988). All too often the dose of a drug is reduced because of a reported 'toxic' level, when the patient is symptom-free and seizure-free. In other patients who are still reporting seizures, the dose may not be increased appropriately for fear of stepping outside the mythical 'therapeutic' range.

Nevertheless, appropriate use of monitoring, preferably on site at the epilepsy clinic (McKee *et al.*, 1992a), can result in improved seizure control with reduced side-effects (McKee *et al.*, 1993). It makes sense to ensure that the drug concentration in a patient with newly diagnosed epilepsy falls within the relevant range to optimize the likelihood of perfect control. Similarly, concentration may be helpful in making the decision whether or not a new clinical problem is a drug side-effect or a red herring. Monitoring can be helpful in patients taking a combination of mutually interacting anticonvulsant agents. Levels are also useful in exploring compliance, as one major reason for therapeutic 'failure' is the inability of a patient to follow the prescribed drug regimen perfectly.

The value of measuring the unbound (free) concentrations is limited to an occasional patient taking a highly bound drug, such as phenytoin, in whom protein binding can be expected to be reduced. Such situations theoretically include late pregnancy, old age, hepatic and renal failure, and the co-prescription of drugs that alter protein binding. Despite the fact that these situations are not uncommon, the evidence supporting the usefulness of free level monitoring is sparse. In addition, the methodology for measuring free levels is more complicated, less reliable and more expensive than assaying total drug concentrations. Saliva sampling will reflect free concentrations of phenytoin, carbamazepine and primidone, but not phenobarbitone or sodium valproate (Thomson and Brodie, 1992).

Information on monitoring the newer anticonvulsant drugs is still incomplete. Vigabatrin acts as an irreversible suicide inhibitor of the catabolic enzyme gamma-aminobutyric acid transaminase. Although its elimination half-life is short, vigabatrin's duration of action exceeds 24 hours, as more enzyme must be synthesized *de novo* (Grant and Heel, 1992). Accordingly, monitoring circulating concentrations of the drug is not helpful in the clinical management of the patient.

Lamotrigine has a half-life of approximately 24 hours, which increases to around 60 hours with administration of sodium valproate and is reduced by 50% in the presence of enzyme-inducing anticonvulsants such as carbamazepine and phenytoin (Brodie, 1992a). Monitoring serum concentrations may, therefore, be of value in tailoring the lamotrigine dose when it is given with other anticonvulsant drugs. Although a tentative target range of 1–4 mg/l has been proposed, population kinetic studies are currently under way in epileptic patients to delineate this further.

Gabapentin has a short half-life of 5–6 hours and does not interact pharmacokinetically with other anticonvulsant drugs (Goa and Sorkin, 1993). In an early study, improvement in seizure control was associated with a linear relationship between gabapentin dose and concentration (Crawford *et al.*, 1987). Also in a major parallel-group, placebo-controlled, add-on trial, gabapentin concentrations were higher in responders than in non-responders (Chadwick, 1990). Although this drug may have potential for monitoring, clarification is still required.

Felbamate has a long half-life of around 20 hours, and there appears to be a linear relationship between the dose and serum concentration (Brodie, 1993). Although experience with the drug is largely limited to studies in which it was added to established therapy in refractory epilepsy, there is some evidence supporting a concentration–effect relationship in patients with Lennox–Gastaut syndrome (Felbamate Study Group in Lennox–Gastaut Syndrome, 1993). Further evaluation of felbamate as monotherapy is required before any conclusions regarding the usefulness of therapeutic drug monitoring can be made.

Oxcarbazepine is a pro-drug which is rapidly converted to the 10-hydroxy metabolite, through which it exerts its clinical effects (Grant and Faulds, 1992). This active moiety has an elimination half-life of around 12 hours, making it a prime target for monitoring serum concentrations. At present, however, there is little evidence in support of a clear-cut relationship between concentration, effect and toxicity. The results of controlled clinical trials, currently under way, may shed some light on this issue.

## CLASSIFICATION OF INTERACTIONS

### Pharmaceutical

Every care is taken to ensure that the ingredients of a drug mixture do not react together chemically, altering their bioavailability or rate of absorption. Despite this, unpredicted mutual interference between compounds can escape initial detection. Changing the filler of phenytoin capsules from lactose to calcium sulphate produced unexpected toxicity (Bochner *et al.*, 1972). Infusing phenytoin in a dextrose solution can lead to precipitation and loss of effect (Kutt, 1989).

### Absorption

Most interactions involving absorption result in a decrease rather than an increase in drug absorption (McInnes and Brodie, 1988). Some drugs form chelates and complexes within the gut, reducing the solubility and absorption of other agents. Reduction in the rate of gastric emptying can decrease the rate of absorption, while more rapid transit time may produce faster, higher peak concentrations. Damage to the gut mucosa can reduce bioavailability of some poorly absorbed compounds. Alteration in gastrointestinal flora by broad-spectrum antibiotics can influence drug absorption by disrupting enterohepatic cycling and reducing bacterial drug conjugation.

Phenytoin absorption can be reduced by several compounds. Antacids form insoluble complexes (Garratt et al., 1979) as do enteral feeding formulae (Bauer, 1982). The same mechanism is probably responsible for the 20% reduction in bioavailability with sucralfate (Smart et al., 1985). Vinblastine, methotrexate and carmustine reduce phenytoin plasma levels by damaging the gut mucosa. Administration of these substances may lead to loss of efficacy (Fincham and Schottelius, 1989; Bollini et al., 1983) and their withdrawal may precipitate toxicity (Bauer, 19982).

Activated charcoal reduces the absorption of carbamazepine and phenobarbitone, probably by sequestering enterically secreted drug (Neuvonen and Elonen, 1980). Cytotoxic drugs, such as adriamycin and cisplatin, also impair carbamazepine absorption by damaging the gut mucosa (Neef and Van der Straaten, 1988). Valproate and phenobarbitone absorption may be limited by concomitant administration of antacids (Hurwitz, 1977), charcoal (Neuvonen et al., 1983) and cytotoxic drugs (Neef and Van der Straaten, 1988).

**Protein binding displacement**

When one drug is displaced from its binding sites on plasma proteins by another there is a transient rise in free concentration, which is almost instantaneously distributed throughout the tissues. A compensatory increase in clearance ensures that the free drug level is similar to that circulating prior to displacement. The total drug concentration falls to accommodate the rise in free fraction. Any alteration in pharmacological effect will be minimal.

The importance of protein binding interactions has been exaggerated from observing circumstances where the displacing drug also caused a degree of inhibition of metabolism. When valproate is given to a patient stabilized on phenytoin, for instance, a marked increase in the free concentration of phenytoin will occur (Mattson et al., 1978) with resultant signs of toxicity in a few susceptible patients (Rodin et al., 1981). This rise is in part caused by a displacement from protein binding sites (Perucca et al., 1980), but the role of inhibition of phenytoin metabolism is much more important (Koch et al., 1981).

Phenylbutazone interacts with phenytoin in a similar manner but the contribution of inhibition is greater than with valproate (Neuvonen et al., 1979). The result is an initial decline in total phenytoin concentrations followed a few days later by an increase to higher levels than occurred previously. Free phenytoin is increased producing signs of toxicity. Similarly, although aspirin displaces valproic acid from its binding sites on plasma proteins, it also inhibits its elimination, resulting occasionally in valproate toxicity (Goulden *et al.*, 1987).

## Drug metabolism

The commonest pharmacokinetic problems with anticonvulsant drugs arise as a consequence of enzyme induction or inhibition. Drug-metabolizing enzymes in the liver are present in multiple forms. There are at least 15 types of cytochrome P450, the oxidative enzyme system most involved in the breakdown of the major anticonvulsant drugs (Ryan and Levin, 1990). Many compounds are biotransformed by more than one type of enzyme, and several enzymes in turn can catalyse the same metabolic step (Perucca, 1987). Accordingly, an interaction is likely to occur only if both drugs bind to the same enzyme system. Adverse effects are also more likely to arise with drugs that are eliminated down a single pathway. Representative lists of clinically significant interactions with established anticonvulsant drugs involving these mechanisms are given in Tables 1–4 (McInnes and Brodie, 1988; Pisani *et al.*, 1990; Brodie, 1992).

## Enzyme induction

Phenytoin, carbamazepine, phenobarbitone and primidone (metabolized in part to phenobarbitone) have the ability to induce the production of oxidative and (to a lesser extent) conjugating enzymes. As protein synthesis is required, the maximum effect is not seen for two to three weeks. The clinical result is increased metabolism of drugs and endogenous hormones with resultant reduction in their circulating concentrations and possible loss of pharmacological effect. Carbamazepine, in addition, can induce its own metabolism to a substantial extent (Rapeport *et al.*, 1983). When an inducer is withdrawn, the process goes into reverse with a decline in the number of enzymes and a gradual increase in the plasma concentration of the induced agent with potential for toxicity. A large number of lipid-soluble drugs are inactivated in the liver and the list of potential interactions is long. Significant deterioration in the patient's clinical state is less likely if the induced drug has a high therapeutic ratio or the extent of enzyme induction is small.

Phenytoin, carbamazepine and phenobarbitone accelerate the elimination of hydrocortisone (Werk *et al.*, 1964; Southern *et al.*, 1969; Choi *et al.*, 1971), dexamethasone (Werk *et al.*, 1969; Haque *et al.*, 1972), prednisolone (Petereit and Meikle, 1977) and methylprednisolone (Stjernholm and Katz, 1975). Clinically significant interactions occur when these enzyme inducers are used

**Table 1.** Clinically significant metabolic interactions involving phenytoin

| | | |
|---|---|---|
| Allopurinol | Enzyme inhibition | Phenytoin toxicity |
| Amiodarone | Enzyme inhibition | Phenytoin toxicity |
| Azapropazone | Enzyme inhibition | Phenytoin toxicity |
| Carbamazepine | Mutual metabolic interference | Increased phenytoin concentration; reduced carbamazepine concentration |
| Chloramphenicol | Enzyme inhibition | Phenytoin toxicity |
| Chlorpromazine | Enzyme inhibition | Phenytoin toxicity |
| Cimetidine | Enzyme inhibition | Phenytoin toxicity |
| Co-trimoxazole | Enzyme inhibition | Phenytoin toxicity |
| Cyclosporin | Enzyme induction | Reduced cyclosporin effect |
| Dexamethasone | Enzyme induction | Reduced steroid effect |
| Diazepam | Enzyme induction | Reduced diazepam effect |
| Disulfiram | Enzyme inhibition | Phenytoin toxicity |
| Ethanol (chronic) | Enzyme induction | Reduced phenytoin effect |
| Fluconazole | Enzyme inhibition | Phenytoin toxicity |
| Hydrocortisone | Enzyme induction | Reduced steroid effect |
| Imipramine | Enzyme inhibition | Phenytoin toxicity |
| Isoniazid | Enzyme inhibition | Phenytoin toxicity |
| Methylprednisolone | Enzyme induction | Loss of steroid effect |
| Metronidazole | Enzyme inhibition | Phenytoin toxicity |
| Mexiletine | Enzyme induction | Reduced mexiletine effect |
| Miconazole | Enzyme inhibition | Phenytoin toxicity |
| Oral contraceptives | Enzyme induction | Contraceptive failure |
| Oxazepam | Enzyme induction | Reduced oxazepam effect |
| Pancuronium | Enzyme induction | Reduced anaesthesia |
| Pethidine | Enzyme induction | Reduced analgesia |
| Phenylbutazone | Enzyme inhibition/ protein binding displacement | Phenytoin toxicity |
| Prednisolone | Enzyme induction | Loss of steroid effect |
| Quinidine | Enzyme induction | Breakthrough arrhythmia |
| Rifampicin | Enzyme induction | Reduced phenytoin concentration |
| Sodium valproate | Enzyme induction Enzyme inhibition/ protein binding displacement | Reduced valproate concentration Phenytoin toxicity |
| Sulphonamides | Enzyme inhibition | Phenytoin toxicity |
| Thioridazine | Enzyme inhibition | Phenytoin toxicity |
| Viloxazine | Enzyme inhibition | Phenytoin toxicity |
| Warfarin | Enzyme induction | Reduced anticoagulation |

in patients taking steroids chronically. Phenobarbitone has been reported to worsen steroid-dependent asthma (Brooks *et al.*, 1972) and reduces the inflammatory response to prednisolone in rheumatoid arthritis (Brooks *et al.*, 1976). Renal allograft survival has been shown to be shorter in individuals treated with phenytoin (Wassner *et al.*, 1976).

**Table 2.**   Clinically significant metabolic interactions involving carbamazepine

| Amitriptyline | Enzyme induction | Reduced amitriptyline effect |
|---|---|---|
| Cimetidine | Enzyme inhibition | Carbamazepine toxicity |
| Clarithromycin | Enzyme inhibition | Carbamazepine toxicity |
| Clonazepam | Enzyme induction | Reduced clonazepam effect |
| Danazol | Enzyme inhibition | Carbamazepine toxicity |
| Dextropropoxyphene | Enzyme inhibition | Carbemazepine toxicity |
| Diltiazem | Enzyme inhibition | Carbamazepine toxicity |
| Doxepin | Enzyme induction | Reduced doxepin effect |
| Erythromycin | Enzyme inhibition | Carbamazepine toxicity |
| Ethosuximide | Enzyme induction | Reduced ethosuximide effect |
| Haloperidol | Enzyme induction | Reduced haloperidol effect |
| Isoniazid | Enzyme inhibition | Carbamazepine toxicity |
| Josamycin | Enzyme inhibition | Carbamazepine toxicity |
| Mianserin | Enzyme induction | Reduced mianserin effect |
| Nomifensine | Enzyme induction | Reduced nomifensine effect |
| Oral contraceptives | Enzyme induction | Contraceptive failure |
| Phenobarbitone | Mutual induction | Decreased concentration of both |
| Phenytoin | Mutual metabolic interference | Increased phenytoin concentration; decreased carbamazepine concentration |
| Primidone | Mutual induction | Decreased concentration of both |
| Sodium valproate | Enzyme induction | Reduced valproate effect |
| | Enzyme inhibition | Carbamazepine toxicity |
| Theophylline | Enzyme induction | Reduced theophylline effect |
| Troleandomycin | Enzyme inhibition | Carbamazepine toxicity |
| Verapamil | Enzyme inhibition | Carbamazepine toxicity |
| Viloxazine | Enzyme inhibition | Carbamazepine toxicity |
| Warfarin | Enzyme induction | Reduced anticoagulation |

**Table 3.**   Clinically significant metabolic interactions involving phenobarbitone and primidone

| Cortisol | Enzyme induction | Loss of steroid effect |
|---|---|---|
| Dextropropoxyphene | Enzyme inhibition | Phenobarbitone toxicity |
| Digitoxin | Enzyme induction | Reduced digitoxin effect |
| Glyceryl trinitrate | Enzyme induction | Reduced nitrate effect |
| Griseofulvin | Enzyme induction | Reduced griseofulvin effect |
| Oral contraceptives | Enzyme induction | Contraceptive failure |
| Rifampicin | Enzyme induction | Increase in seizure frequency |
| Sodium valproate | Enzyme inhibition | Phenobarbitone toxicity |
| Testosterone | Enzyme induction | Reduced steroid effect |
| Tricyclic antidepressants | Enzyme induction | Breakthrough depression |
| Warfarin | Enzyme induction | Reduced anticoagulation |

**Table 4.**  Clinically significant metabolic interactions involving sodium valproate

| | | |
|---|---|---|
| Amitriptyline | Enzyme inhibition | Tricyclic toxicity |
| Aspirin | Enzyme inhibition/protein binding displacement | Valproate toxicity |
| Carbamazepine | Enzyme induction | Reduced valproate concentration |
| | Enzyme inhibition | Carbamazepine toxicity |
| Diazepam | Enzyme inhibition/protein binding displacement | Increased diazepam effect |
| Ethosuximide | Enzyme inhibition | Increased ethosuximide effect |
| Phenobarbitone | Enzyme inhibition | Increased phenobarbitone effect |
| Phenytoin | Enzyme induction | Reduced valproate concentration |
| | Enzyme inhibition/protein binding displacement | Phenytoin toxicity |

Increased episodes of breakthrough bleeding and contraceptive failure have been reported among patients treated with enzyme-inducing anti-convulsant drugs who are also dependent on the oral contraceptive pill (Matt-son *et al.*, 1986). Prescribing a formulation containing a high dose of eth-inyloestradiol is now standard practice. Some patients, particularly those taking carbamazepine, may need to take as much as 100 µg of oestrogen daily to prevent breakthrough bleeding.

**Enzyme inhibition**

Most inhibitory reactions involve competition between two protagonists for the same binding sites on hepatic mono-oxygenase enzymes (McInnes and Brodie, 1988). This produces an increase in plasma level of the inhibited drug, maximal five half-lives later when a new steady state is achieved. The extent of the interaction and, therefore, of the clinical effect varies among individ-uals and is consequently unpredictable. It depends to some extent on the dose (and concentration) of the inhibitor (McKee *et al.*, 1992b). Potentiation occurs quickly for drugs with short half-lives and more slowly for those eliminated less efficiently. Commonly prescribed enzyme inhibitors include ery-thromycin, cimetidine and dextropropoxyphene (Table 5). Sodium valproate inhibits metabolic enzymes, but clinical problems seem to occur largely in patients receiving other anticonvulsant drugs (Levy and Koch, 1982). When an inhibitory drug is withdrawn, the concentration of the target drug will fall with possible attenuation of its pharmacological effect (Brodie, 1992b).

Inhibition of phenytoin metabolism is more likely to be clinically significant than with other anticonvulsant drugs owing to its saturable kinetics (Richens

**Table 5.**   Some enzyme inhibitors in clinical use

| | |
|---|---|
| Allopurinol | Metronidazole |
| Amiodarone | Miconazole |
| Azapropazone | Nortriptyline |
| Chloramphenicol | Omeprazole |
| Chlorpromazine | Oral contraceptives |
| Cimetidine | Oxyphenbutazone |
| Ciprofloxacin | Perphenazine |
| Danazol | Phenylbutazone |
| Dextropropoxyphene | Primaquine |
| Diltiazem | Propafenone |
| Dilsulfiram | Propranolol |
| Ethanol (acute) | Quinidine |
| Erythromycin | Sodium valproate |
| Fluconazole | Sulphinpyrazone |
| Fluvoxamine | Sulphonamides |
| Imipramine | Thioridazine |
| Isoniazid | Trimethoprim |
| Ketoconazole | Verapamil |
| Metoprolol | Viloxazine |

and Warrington, 1979). For example, giving isoniazid (Miller *et al.*, 1979), dextropropoxyphene (Kutt, 1989), phenothiazines (Vincent, 1980) and cimetidine (Frigo *et al.*, 1983) will produce a marked rise in phenytoin concentration in many patients, some of whom will develop manifestations of toxicity (Vincent, 1980). Carbamazepine too is particularly susceptible to clinically significant inhibitory interactions as a consequence of autoinduction of its metabolism (Macphee and Brodie, 1985). Such interactions have been reported with dextropropoxyphene (Dam *et al.*, 1977), erythromycin (Wong *et al.*, 1983; Carranco *et al.*, 1985), cimetidine (Macphee *et al.*, 1984) and danazol (Kramer *et al.*, 1986). The calcium antagonists, verapamil and diltiazem, increase carbamazepine levels on average by 50% and may produce symptoms of neurotoxicity (Brodie and Macphee, 1986; Macphee *et al.*, 1986). Dextropropoxyphene also inhibits the metabolism of phenobarbitone (Hansen *et al.*, 1980).

## MUTUAL PHARMACOKINETIC INTERACTIONS BETWEEN ANTICONVULSANT DRUGS

Pharmacokinetic interactions between anticonvulsant drugs are common and unpredictable. All enzyme inducers will accelerate the breakdown of sodium valproate, ethosuximide and the benzodiazepines, clonazepam and clobazam (Pisani *et al.*, 1990). A complex interaction results when phenytoin and carbamazepine are given together. The metabolism of the latter can be induced by the former, whereas the latter inhibits the elimination of the former by competing for binding sites on the same population of metabolic enzymes (Zielinski and Haidukewych, 1987). This results in a rise in phenytoin and a fall in carbamazepine concentrations when one or other is introduced (Browne *et al.*, 1988). The opposite prevails when either drug is withdrawn.

Interactions involving carbamazepine are further complicated by the presence of an active metabolite, carbamazepine 10,11-epoxide, which is itself broken down by epoxide hydrolase to the inert dihydrodiol. Carbamazepine epoxide possesses anticonvulsant activity (Tomson *et al.*, 1990) and has been implicated in some of the neurotoxic side-effects associated with the drug (Patsalos *et al.*, 1985; Gillham *et al.*, 1988; McKee *et al.*, 1989). Higher epoxide levels occur in epileptic patients taking carbamazepine in combination with phenytoin, sodium valproate and phenobarbitone (Brodie *et al.*, 1983) compared with monotherapy. The former two drugs induce its formation (Brodie *et al.*, 1983), while valproate inhibits its breakdown (Macphee *et al.*, 1988) in an unpredictable way (McKee *et al.*, 1992b).

## INTERACTIONS INVOLVING NEW ANTICONVULSANT DRUGS

The efficacy of potential anticonvulsant compounds is routinely assessed by adding them to existing treatment in patients with refractory epilepsy. Pharmacokinetic interactions may result that mask the therapeutic effect of the novel agent and hence slow its development. Such problems can be anticipated if the metabolic characteristics and concentration-related side-effects of the new drug are known. Pharmacokinetic parameters for drugs discussed in this chapter are outlined in Table 6. Similar data for established anticonvulsant drugs have been published elsewhere (Brodie, 1990).

### Vigabatrin

*Non-anticonvulsant drug interactions*

As would be expected from its kinetic profile, vigabatrin excretion is largely unaffected by concomitant medication and no interactions have been reported to date (Grant and Heel, 1991). The drug itself has no effect on hepatic metabolic processes.

*Anticonvulsant drug interactions*

Most of the information regarding the effect of vigabatrin on established anticonvulsant medication has been derived from measurement of concomitant drug levels during placebo-controlled trials. The drug has no effect on concentrations of carbamazepine or sodium valproate (Rimmer and Richens,

**Table 6.** Pharmacokinetics of some new anticonvulsant drugs

| Drug | Absorption (bioavailability) | Distribution volume (l/kg) | Protein binding (% bound) | Elimination half-life (hours) | Route(s) of elimination | Comments |
|---|---|---|---|---|---|---|
| Vigabatrin | Rapid (60–85%) | 0.6–1.0 | 0 | 5–7 | Largely excreted unchanged | Long-acting owing to irreversible binding to GABA transaminase |
| Lamotrigine | Rapid (95–100%) | 0.8–1.2 | 55 | 22–36 | Hepatic metabolism to glucuronide conjugate | Metabolism induced or inhibited by other anticonvulsant drugs |
| Gabapentin | Rapid (50–60%) | 0.8–1.0 | 0 | 5–7 | Largely excreted unchanged | Limited absorption at high dosage |
| Felbamate | Rapid (> 90%) | 0.76–0.81 | 30 | 14–23 | Partly metabolized and partly excreted unchanged | Mutual metabolic interference with other anticonvulsant drugs |
| Oxcarbazepine* | Rapid (> 90%) | 0.7–0.8 | 40 | 8–10 | Undergoes reduction to active metabolite which is excreted as glucuronide conjugate | Acts through active metabolite |

*Data for active metabolite.

1984; Gram et al., 1985; Pedersen et al., 1985; Loiseau et al., 1986). In an open study, Browne et al. (1987) noted 7% and 11% decreases in phenobarbitone and primidone levels respectively in patients receiving additional vigabatrin. These were not accompanied by any alteration in the patients' clinical status. No change has been noted in clonazepam (Pedersen et al., 1985; Matilainen et al., 1988), clobazam (Luna et al., 1989), ethosuximide or oxcarbazepine (Pedersen et al., 1985) levels during co-administration of vigabatrin.

A 20% decrease in serum phenytoin concentrations has been observed during vigabatrin treatment (Rimmer and Richens, 1984). Deterioration in seizure control has been attributed to a fall in phenytoin concentrations, however, in only one patient (Browne *et al.*, 1987). This interaction has been explored further by Rimmer and Richens (1989), but the underlying mechanism remains unclear. The reduction in phenytoin concentration occurred after four weeks' treatment with 3 g vigabatrin daily. No alteration in hepatic metabolism or protein binding was observed. Phenytoin absorption has also been reported to be unaffected by vigabatrin administration (Gatti *et al.*, 1993). When vigabatrin is prescribed in a patient taking phenytoin, it may be advisable to measure the serum phenytoin level to anticipate the need for a small increment in dose. More importantly, withdrawal of vigabatrin therapy in a patient stabilized on both drugs may result in phenytoin toxicity.

## Lamotrigine

### Non-anticonvulsant drug interactions

Lamotrigine has little effect on the metabolism of other agents. It does not induce or inhibit hepatic metabolic enzymes (Goa *et al.*, 1993). However, paracetamol has been reported to induce lamotrigine's metabolism (Depot *et al.*, 1990). The mechanism of this interaction is unknown, as is its clinical relevance.

### Anticonvulsant drug interactions

Concomitant administration of other anticonvulsant drugs has a profound effect on lamotrigine's metabolism (Brodie, 1990). Enzyme inducers reduce its half-life from a mean of 29 hours to 15 hours (Binnie *et al.*, 1986; Jawad *et al.*, 1987). Sodium valproate lengthens it to 60 hours, probably by inhibiting hepatic glucuronidation, its major pathway of elimination (Yuen *et al.*, 1992). If valproate is taken in combination with an enzyme inducer, the half-life of lamotrigine is likely to be around 24 hours. In practice, it is unlikely that any problems will be encountered when lamotrigine is introduced, as the dose will be titrated against therapeutic effect. This is not the case when anticonvulsant drugs are discontinued. Withdrawal of valproate will cause lamotrigine levels to fall substantially. Conversely, when an enzyme inducer is discontinued, the lamotrigine concentration can be expected to rise.

There have been reports of symptoms of neurotoxicity (headache, nausea, dizziness, diplopia, ataxia) in patients taking carbamazepine in whom lamotrigine has been introduced (Wolf, 1992). These symptoms disappear when the dose of either drug is reduced. The suggestion from an open study that carbamazepine epoxide levels are elevated by lamotrigine (Warner *et al.*, 1992) has not been supported by results from a recent placebo-controlled, dose-ranging trial of additional lamotrigine in patients with refractory epilepsy (Stolarek *et al.*, 1993). This, therefore, is likely to be a pharmacodynamic rather than a pharmacokinetic interaction.

## Gabapentin

*Non-anticonvulsant drug interactions*

As gabapentin is excreted unchanged by the kidney, it is perhaps not surprising that there are few reports of interactions with other medicaments. The aluminium/magnesium antacid, Maalox, caused a small (20%) reduction in gabapentin bioavailability (Busch *et al.*, 1992). Cimetidine has been observed to reduce gabapentin renal clearance by 12% (Busch *et al.*, 1993). Neither interaction is likely to be of clinical significance. Gabapentin does not alter the pharmacokinetics of ethinyloestradiol (Busch *et al.*, 1993).

*Anticonvulsant drug interactions*

Gabapentin does not interact with nor is it influenced kinetically by phenytoin, carbamazepine (Goa and Sorkin, 1993), sodium valproate (Basim *et al.*, 1990) or phenobarbitone (Hooper *et al.*, 1991).

## Felbamate

*Non-anticonvulsant drug interactions*

Although felbamate may be an enzyme inducer or inhibitor (Segelman *et al.*, 1985; Swinyard *et al.*, 1987) and, therefore, has the potential to interfere with the metabolism of other drugs, no interactions with non-anticonvulsant medication have been explored to date (Brodie, 1993). Such studies are urgently awaited.

*Anticonvulsant drug interactions*

Most of the information regarding interactions with felbamate and other anticonvulsant drugs has been generated in the course of clinical trials (Palmer and McTavish, 1993). The addition of felbamate results in an increase in serum phenytoin levels with the production of neurotoxicity (Milne and Pledger, 1987; Fuerst *et al.*, 1988). This interaction occurred without a change in phenytoin protein binding (Feurst *et al.*, 1988). As both drugs undergo hydroxylation in the liver, felbamate has been suggested to act as a competitive inhibitor of phenytoin metabolism (Feurst *et al.*, 1988).

Carbamazepine concentrations fell by 10–40% with additional felbamate in epileptic patients (Holmes *et al.*, 1987; Feurst *et al.*, 1988; Graves *et al.*, 1989; Albani *et al.*, 1991). This was accompanied, however, by a 26–51% increase in levels of the active metabolite, carbamazepine epoxide (Graves *et al.*, 1989; Albani *et al.*, 1991). As this interaction occurred without change in carbamazepine's free fraction, it is likely that felbamate induced carbamazepine metabolism (Graves *et al.*, 1989; Albani *et al.*, 1991). As the epoxide also has anticonvulsant activity (Tomson *et al.*, 1990), the overall clinical significance of this interaction is unclear.

Felbamate administration decreased the clearance of valproate with an associated increase in circulating concentrations in epileptic patients (Wagner *et al.*, 1991a). No change in protein binding was observed, and so the drug can be assumed to inhibit valproate metabolism. It may, therefore, be necessary to reduce the dose of valproate when adding felbamate to the therapeutic regimen.

Established anticonvulsant drugs, in turn, influence the pharmacokinetics of felbamate. In an open study, felbamate concentrations were higher in patients treated with valproate than in those taking carbamazepine or phenytoin (Wagner *et al.*, 1990). Similarly, reductions in carbamazepine and phenytoin dosage produced a 34% fall in felbamate clearance (Wagner *et al.*, 1991b). These data suggest that enzyme-inducing anticonvulsant drugs increase felbamate metabolism, while valproate may inhibit it. This has importance too for patients taking felbamate, in whom one of these anticonvulsant drugs is discontinued.

## Oxcarbazepine

*Non-anticonvulsant drug interactions*

Oxcarbazepine has less potential than carbamazepine to induce liver enzymes and so influence the metabolism of other drugs (Grant and Faulds, 1992). Unlike carbamazepine, it does not alter the markers of enzyme induction, such as antipyrine clearance and urinary 6-beta-hydrocortisol excretion (Larkin *et al.*, 1991b). Volunteer studies have suggested it does not interfere with warfarin metabolism (Kramer *et al.*, 1992), nor will cimetidine (Keranen *et al.*, 1992) or dextropoxyphene (Morgensen *et al.*, 1992) inhibit its breakdown as is the case with carbamazepine (Baciewicz, 1986). However, decreased bioavailability of the oral contraceptive pill has been noted in some patients treated with oxcarbazepine (Klosterkov-Jensen *et al.*, 1992). In addition, the area under the concentration–time curve of the calcium antagonist felodipine was reduced by 28% following the introduction of oxcarbazepine (Zaccara *et al.*, 1993) compared with a 90% reduction in similar studies with carbamazepine, phenytoin and phenobarbitone (Capewell *et al.*, 1987, 1988). It has been suggested that at high doses oxcarbazepine can act as an enzyme inducer (Patsalos *et al.*, 1990). An alternative and more likely hypothesis is that the drug selectively induces a single isoform of cytochrome P450, namely IIIA (Grant and Faulds, 1992).

*Anticonvulsant drug interactions*

Treatment with oxcarbazepine has not resulted in autoinduction of metabolism (Larkin *et al.*, 1991b). In patients changed from carbamazepine to oxcarbazepine, steady state plasma concentrations of phenytoin and valproate rose by 20–30% (Bulau *et al.*, 1987; Houtkooper *et al.*, 1987). This also suggests that the new agent is a less powerful inducer than carbamazepine with reduced potential for interactions with other anticonvulsant drugs.

These observations have been confirmed in a placebo-controlled study exploring the interaction of oxcarbazepine with carbamazepine, phenytoin and valproate in epileptic patients taking one of these first-line agents as monotherapy (McKee *et al.*, 1994). Oxcarbazepine had little effect on the areas under the concentration–time curve of concomitant anticonvulsant medication, suggesting an absence of important metabolic interference with these agents. However, the areas under the concentration–time curve of the active metabolite, hydroxycarbazepine, were lower in patients taking carbamazepine and, to a lesser extent, phenytoin than in controls. This would be consistent with a small induction effect, which would have little clinical relevance, as titration of the oxcarbazepine dose would be the normal course of events. However, withdrawal of either drug might produce a rise in hydroxycarbazepine concentrations sufficient, perhaps, to produce concentration-related side-effects in a susceptible patient. Enzyme induction with phenobarbitone has also been shown to decrease the area under the concentration–time curve of hydroxycarbazepine following a single dose of oxcarbazepine (Tartara *et al.*, 1993). Co-medication with clobazam does not appear to influence the metabolism of oxcarbazepine (Arnoldussen *et al.*, 1993).

## CONCLUSION

The introduction of new anticonvulsant drugs is necessary to offer hope to the large minority of patients with refractory epilepsy. This will result inevitably in many patients taking a combination of medicines, some of which will produce pharmacokinetic interactions. With the newer agents, therapeutic drug monitoring will not be helpful, as the relationships of concentration, effect and toxicity will not be defined at such an early stage. An appreciation of the pharmacokinetics of the drugs and the mechanisms likely to lead to a significant interaction will enable the clinician to anticipate problems and allow the formulation of a safe management plan. In the final analysis, the clinical state of the patient will dictate whether an adverse interaction produces a genuine clinical problem.

## ACKNOWLEDGEMENT

The authors' grateful thanks go to Mrs Moya Dewar for her expert secretarial assistance.

## REFERENCES

Albani F, Theodore WH, Washington P, Devinsky O, Bromfield E, Porter RJ and Nice EJ (1991) Effect of felbamate on plasma levels of carbamazepine and its metabolites. *Epilepsia,* **32**, 130–132.

Arnoldussen W, Hulsman J and Rentmeester T (1993) Interaction of valproate and clobazam on the metabolism of oxcarbazepine. *Epilepsia,* **34**, (Suppl. 2) 160.

Baciewicz AM (1986) Carbamazepine drug interactions. *Ther. Drug Monit.,* **8**, 305–317.

Basim M, Uthman EI, Hammond EJ and Wilder BJ (1990) Absence of gabapentin and valproate interaction: an evoked potential and pharmacokinetic study. *Epilepsia,* **31**, 645.

Bauer LA (1982) Interference of oral phenytoin absorption by continuous nasogastric feedings. *Neurology,* **32**, 570–572.

Binnie CD, van Emde Boas W, Kasteleijn-Nolste-Trenite DGA *et al.* (1986) Acute effects of lamotrigine (BW430C) in persons with epilepsy. *Epilepsia,* **27**, 248–254.

Bochner F, Hooper WD, Tyrer JH and Eadie MJ (1972) Factors involved in an outbreak of phenytoin intoxication. *J. Neurol. Sci,* **16**, 481–487.

Bollini P, Riva R, Albani F, Ida N, Cacciari L, Bollini C and Baruzzi A (1983) Decreased phenytoin level during antineoplastic therapy: a case report. *Epilepsia,* **24**, 75–78.

Brodie MJ (1990) Established anticonvulsants and the treatment of refractory epilepsy. *Lancet,* **336**, 350–354.

Brodie MJ (1992a) Lamotrigine. *Lancet,* **339**, 1397–1400.

Brodie MJ (1992b) Drug interactions and epilepsy. *Epilepsia,* **33**, (suppl. 1), S13–S22.

Brodie MJ (1993) Felbamate: a new antiepileptic drug. *Lancet,* **341**, 1445–1446.

Brodie MJ and Feely J (1988) Practical clinical pharmacology. Therapeutic drug monitoring and clinical trials. *Br. Med. J.,* **296**, 1110–1114.

Brodie MJ and Macphee GJA (1986) Carbamazepine neurotoxicity precipitated by diltiazem. *Br. Med. J.,* **292**, 1170–1171.

Brodie MJ, Forrest GD and Rapeport WG (1983) Carbamazepine 10,11 epoxide concentrations in epileptics on carbamazepine alone and in combination with other anticonvulsants. *Br. J. Clin. Pharmacol.,* **16**, 747–750.

Brooks SM, Werk EE, Ackerman SJ, Sullivan I and Thrasher K (1972) Adverse effects of phenobarbital on corticosteroid metabolism in patients with bronchial asthma. *N. Eng. J. Med.,* **286**, 1125–1128.

Brooks PM, Buchanan WW, Grove M and Downie NW (1976) Effects of enzyme induction on metabolism of prednisolone: clinical and laboratory study. *Ann. Rheum. Dis.,* **35**, 339–343.

Browne TR, Mattson RH, Penry JK *et al.* (1987) Vigabatrin for refractory complex partial seizures: multicentre single-blind study with long-term follow-up. *Neurology,* **37**, 184–189.

Browne TR, Szabo BK, Evans JG, Evans BA, Greenblatt DJ and Mikati MA (1988) Carbamazepine increases phenytoin serum concentration and reduces phenytoin clearance. *Neurology*, **38**, 1146–1150.

Bulau P, Stoll KD and Froscher W (1987) Oxcarbazepine versus carbamazepine. In: *Advances in Epilepsy* (eds P Woy, M Dam, D Janz and F Dreifuss), Vol. 16, pp. S31–36. Raven Press, New York.

Busch JA, Radulovic LL, Bockbrader HN, Underwood BA, Sedman AJ and Chang T (1992) Effect of Maalox TC on single-dose pharmacokinetics of gabapentin capsules in healthy subjects. *Pharm. Res.*, **9**, 315.

Busch J, Bockbrader HN, Randinitis EJ *et al.* (1993) Lack of clinically significant drug interactions with Neurontin (gabapentin). *Epilepsia*, **34**, (suppl. 2), 158.

Capewell S, Freestone S, Critchley JAJH, Pottage A and Prescott LF (1987) Gross reduction in felodipine bioavailability in patients taking anticonvulsants. *Br. J. Clin. Pharmacol.*, **24**, 243–244.

Capewell S, Freestone S, Critchley JAJH and Pottage A (1988) Reduced felodipine bioavailability in patients taking anticonvulsants. *Lancet*, **ii**, 480–482.

Carranco E, Karens J, Schenby C, Peak V and Ar-Rayeh S (1985) Carbamazepine toxicity induced by concurrent erythromycin therapy. *Arch. Neurol.*, **42**, 187–188.

Chadwick D (1990) Gabapentin in partial epilepsy. *Lancet*, **335**, 1114–1117.

Choi Y, Thrasher K, Werk EE, Sholiton LJ and Ounger C (1971) Effect of diphenylhydantoin on cortisol kinetics in humans. *J. Pharmacol. Exp. Therap.*, **176**, 27–34.

Crawford P, Ghadiali E, Lane R, Blumhardt L and Chadwick D (1987) Gabapentin as an antiepileptic drug in man. *J. Neurol. Neurosurg. Psychiatry*, **50**, 682–686.

Dam M, Kristiansen CB, Hansen BS and Christiansen J (1977) Interaction between carbamazepine and propoxyphene in man. *Acta Neurol. Scand.*, **56**, 603–607.

Depot M, Powell JR, Messenheumer JA, Cloutier G and Dalton MJ (1990) Kinetic effects of multiple oral doses of acetaminophen on a single oral dose of lamotrigine. *Clin. Pharmacol. Therap.*, **48**, 346–355.

Felbamate Study Group in Lennox–Gastaut Syndrome (1993) Efficacy of felbamate in childhood epileptic encephalopathy (Lennox–Gastaut syndrome). *N. Eng. J. Med.*, **328**, 29–33.

Fincham RW and Schottelius DD (1979) Decreased phenytoin levels in antineoplastic therapy. *Ther. Drug Monit.*, **1**, 277–283.

Frigo GM, Lecchini S, Caravaggi M *et al.* (1983) Reduction in phenytoin clearance caused by cimetidine. *Eur. J. Clin. Pharmac.*, **25**, 135–137.

Fuerst RH, Graves NM, Leppik IE, Brundage RC, Holmes GB and Remmel RP (1988) Felbamate increases phenytoin but decreases carbamazepine concentrations. *Epilepsia*, **29**, 488–491.

Garratt WR, Carter BL and Pellock JM (1979) Bioavailability of phenytoin administered with antacids. *Ther. Drug Monit.*, **1**, 435–437.

Gatti G, Bartoli A, Marchiselli R *et al.* (1993) Gamma vinyl GABA (vigabatrin) does not affect gastrointestinal absorption of phenytoin in epileptic patients. *Epilepsia*, **34** (suppl. 2), 120.

Gillham RA, Williams N, Weidmann K, Butler E, Larkin JG and Brodie MJ (1988) Concentration–effect relationships with carbamazepine and its epoxide on psychomotor and cognitive function in epileptic patients. *J. Neurol. Neurosurg. Psychiatry*, **51**, 929–933.

Goa KL and Sorkin EM (1993) Gabapentin: a review of its pharmacological properties and clinical potential in epilepsy. *Drugs*, **46**, 409–427.

Goa KL, Ross SL and Chrisp P (1993) Lamotrigine: a review of its pharmacological properties and clinical efficacy in epilepsy. *Drugs*, **46**, 152–176.

Goulden KJ, Dooley JM, Camfield PR and Fraser AD (1987) Clinical valproate toxicity induced by acetylsalicyclic acid. *Neurology,* **37**, 1392–1394.

Gram L, Klosterkov-Jensen P and Dam M (1985) Gamma-vinyl GABA: a double-blind, placebo-controlled trial in partial epilepsy. *Ann. Neurol.,* **16**, 262–266.

Grant SM and Faulds D (1992) Oxcarbazepine: a review of its pharmacology and therapeutic potential in epilepsy, trigeminal neuralgia and affective disorders. *Drugs,* **42**, 873–888.

Grant SM and Heel RC (1991) Vigabatrin. *Drugs,* **41**, 889–926.

Graves NM, Holmes GB, Fuerst GB and Leppik IE (1989) Effect of felbamate on phenytoin and carbamazepine serum concentrations. *Epilepsia,* **30**, 225–229.

Hansen BS, Dam M, Brandt J *et al.* (1980) Influence of dextropropoxyphene on steady-state serum levels and protein binding of three antiepileptic drugs. *Acta Neurol. Scand.,* **61**, 357–367.

Hague N, Thrasher K, Werk EE, Knowles MC and Sholiton LJ (1972) Studies on dexamethasone metabolism in man: effect of diphenylhydantoin. *J. Clin. Endocrinol. Met.,* **34**, 44–50.

Holmes GB, Graves NM, Leppik IE and Fuerst KH (1987) Felbamate: bidirectional effects on phenytoin and carbamazepine serum concentrations. *Epilepsia,* **28**, 578–579.

Hooper WD, Kavanagh MC, Herkis GK and Eadie MJ (1991) Lack of pharmacokinetic interaction between phenobarbital and gabapentin. *Br. J. Clin. Pharmac.,* **31**, 171–174.

Houtkooper MA, Lammertsma A, Meijer JWA *et al.* (1987) Oxcarbazepine (GPF1680): a possible alternative to carbamazepine. *Epilepsia,* **25**, 693–698.

Hurwitz A (1977) Antacid therapy and drug kinetics. *Clin. Pharmacokinet.,* **2**, 269–280.

Jawad S, Yuen WC, Peck AW, Hamilton MJ, Oxley JR and Richens A (1987) Lamotrigine: single-dose pharmacokinetics and initial one week experience in refractory epilepsy. *Epilepsy Res.,* **1**, 194–201.

Keranen T, Jolkkonen J, Klosterkov-Jensen P and Menge GP (1992) Oxcarbazepine does not interact with cimetidine in healthy volunteers. *Acta Neurol. Scand.,* **85**, 239–242.

Klosterkov-Jensen P, Saano V, Harling P, Svenstrup B and Menge GP (1992) Possible interaction between oxcarbazepine and an oral contraceptive. *Epilepsia,* **33**, 1149–1152.

Koch KM, Ludwick BT and Levy RH (1981) Phenytoin-valproic acid interaction in rhesus monkey. *Epilepsia,* **22**, 19–25.

Kramer G, Theisohn M, Von Unruh GE and Eichelbaum M (1986) Carbamazepine-danazol interaction: its mechanism examined by a stable isotope technique. *Ther. Drug Monit.,* **8**, 387–392.

Kramer G, Tettenborn B, Klosterkov-Jensen B, Menge GP and Stoll KD (1992) Oxcarbazepine does not affect the anticoagulant activity of warfarin. *Epilepsia,* **33**, 1145–1148.

Kutt H (1989) Phenytoin. Interactions with other drugs. In: *Antiepileptic Drugs,* 3rd edn (eds R. Levy, R Mattson, B Meldrum, JK Penry and FE Dreifuss), pp. 215–232. Raven Press, New York.

Larkin JG, Herrick AL, McGuire GM, Percy-Robb I and Brodie MJ (1991a) Antiepileptic drug monitoring at the epilepsy clinic: a prospective evaluation. *Epilepsia,* **32**, 89–95.

Larkin JG, McKee PJW, Forrest G *et al.* (1991b) Lack of enzyme induction with oxcarbazepine (600mg daily) in healthy subjects. *Br. J. Clin. Pharmacol.,* **31**, 65–71.

Levy RH and Koch KM (1982) Drug interactions with valproic acid. *Drugs,* **24,** 543–556.

Loiseau P, Hardenberg JP, Pistre M, Euyot M, Schechter PJ and Tell GP (1986) Double-blind, placebo-controlled study of vigabatrin (gamma-vinyl GABA) in drug-resistant epilepsy. *Epilepsia,* **27,** 115–120.

Luna D, Dulac O, Pajot N and Beaumont D (1989) Vigabatrin in the treatment of childhood epilepsies: a single-blind placebo-controlled study. *Epilepsia,* **30,** 430–437.

Macphee GJA and Brodie MJ (1985) Carbamazepine substitution in severe partial epilepsy: implication of autoinduction of metabolism. *Postgrad. Med. J.,* **61,** 779–783.

Macphee GJA, McInnes GT, Thompson GG and Brodie MJ (1986) Verapamil potentiates carbamazepine neurotoxicity: a clinically important inhibitory interaction. *Lancet,* **i,** 700–703.

Macphee GJA, Thompson GG, Scobie G *et al.* (1984) Effect of cimetidine on carbamazepine auto- and hetero-induction in man. *Br. J. Clin. Pharmacol.,* **18,** 411–419.

Macphee GJA, Mitchell J, Wiseman L, McLellan AR, Park BK, McInnes GT and Brodie MJ (1988) Effect of sodium valproate on carbamazepine disposition and psychomotor profile in man. *Br. J. Clin. Pharmac.,* **25,** 59–66.

Matilainen R, Pitkinen A, Ruutianen T, Mervaala E and Sarlund H (1988) Effect of vigabatrin on epilepsy in mentally retarded patients: a 7 month follow-up study. *Neurology,* **38,** 743–747.

Mattson RH, Cramer JA, Williamson PC and Novelly RA (1978) Valproic acid in epilepsy: clinical and pharmacological effects. *Ann. Neurol.,* **3,** 20–25.

Mattson RH, Cramer JA, Darney PD and Naftolin F (1986) Use of oral contraceptives by women with epilepsy. *JAMA,* **256,** 238–240.

McInnes GT and Brodie MJ (1988) Drug interactions that matter. A critical reappraisal. *Drugs,* **36,** 83–110.

McKee PJW, Larkin JG and Brodie MJ (1989) Acute psychosis with carbamazepine and sodium valproate. *Lancet,* **i,** 167.

McKee PJW, Percy-Robb I and Brodie MJ (1992a) Therapeutic drug monitoring improves seizure control and reduces anticonvulsant side-effects in patients with refractory epilepsy. *Seizure,* **1,** 275–279.

McKee PJW, Blacklaw J, Butler E, Gillham RA and Brodie MJ (1992b) Variability and clinical relevance of the interaction between sodium valproate and carbamazepine in epileptic patients. *Epilepsy Res.,* **11,** 193–198.

McKee PJW, Larkin JG, Brodie A, Percy-Robb I and Brodie MJ (1993) Five years of anticonvulsant monitoring on site at the epilepsy clinic. *Ther. Drug Monit.,* **15,** 83–90.

McKee PJW, Blacklaw J, Forrest G *et al.* (1994) A double-blind, placebo-controlled interaction study between oxcarbazepine and carbamazepine, sodium valproate and phenytoin in epileptic patients. *Br. J. Clin. Pharmacol.,* **37,** 27–34.

Neef C and Van der Straaten (1988) An interaction between cytostatic and anticonvulsant drugs. *Clin. Pharmacol. Therap.,* **43,** 372–375.

Neuvonen PJ and Elonen E (1980) Effect of activated charcoal on absorption and elimination of phenobarbitone, carbamazepine and phenylbutazone in man. *Eur. J. Clin. Pharmac.,* **17,** 51–57.

Neuvonen PJ, Lehtovaara R, Bardy A and Elonen E (1979) Antipyrine analgesic in patients on antiepileptic drug therapy. *Eur. J. Clin. Pharmac.,* **15,** 263–268.

Neuvonen PJ, Kannisto H and Hirvisalo EL (1983) Effect of activated charcoal on absorption of tolbutamide and valproate in man. *Eur. J. Clin. Pharmac.,* **24,** 243–246.

Palmer KJ and McTavish DS (1993) Felbamate: a review of its pharmacodynamic and pharmacokinetic properties and therapeutic efficacy in epilepsy. *Drugs*, **45**, 1041–1065.

Patsalos PN, Stephenson TJ, Krishna S, Elyas AA, Lascelles PT and Wiles CM (1985) Side-effects induced by carbamazepine 10,11 epoxide. *Lancet*, **ii**, 496.

Patsalos PN, Zakrzewska JM and Elyas AA (1990) Dose dependent enzyme induction by oxcarbazepine. *Eur. J. Clin. Pharmac.*, **39**, 187–188.

Pedersen SA, Klosterkov P, Gram L and Dam M (1985) Long-term study of gamma-vinyl GABA in the treatment of epilepsy. *Acta Neurol. Scand.*, **72**, 295–298.

Perucca E (1987) Clinical implications of hepatic microsomal enzyme induction by antiepileptic drugs. *Pharmacol. Ther.*, **33**, 139–144.

Perucca E, Hebdige S, Frigo MD, Gatti G, Lecchini S and Crema A (1980) Interaction between phenytoin and valproic acid: plasma protein binding and metabolic effects. *Clin. Pharmacol. Therap.*, **28**, 779–789.

Petereil LB and Meikle AW (1977) Effectiveness of prednisolone during phenytoin therapy. *Clin. Pharmacol. Therap.*, **22**, 912–916.

Petrie JC and Cluff LE (1980) Evaluation of drug interactions. In: *Clinically Important Adverse Drug Interactions*, Vol. 1, *Cardiovascular and Respiratory Disease Therapy* (ed. JC Petrie), pp. 1–5. Elsevier, Amsterdam.

Pisani F, Perucca E and Di Perri R (1990) Clinically relevant antiepileptic drug interactions. *J. Int. Med. Res.*, **18**, 1–15.

Rapeport WG, McInnes GT, Thompson GG, Forrest G, Park BK and Brodie MJ (1983) Hepatic enzyme induction and leucocyte delta aminolaevulinic acid synthetase activity: studies with carbamazepine. *Br. J. Clin. Pharmacol.*, **16**, 133–137.

Richens A and Warrington S (1979) When should plasma drug levels be monitored? *Drugs*, **17**, 488–500.

Rimmer EM and Richens A (1984) Double-blind study of gamma vinyl GABA in patients with refractory epilepsy. *Lancet*, **i**, 189–190.

Rimmer EM and Richens A (1989) Interaction between vigabatrin and phenytoin. *Br. J. Clin. Pharmacol.*, **27**, 27S–33S.

Rodin EA, De Sousa G, Haidukewyck D, Lodhi R and Berchou RC (1981) Dissociation between free and bound phenytoin levels in the presence of valproic acid. *Arch. Neurol.*, **38**, 240–242.

Ryan DE and Levin W (1990) Purification and characterization of hepatic microsomal cytochrome P-450. *Pharmacol. Ther.*, **45**, 153–239.

Segelman FH, Kelton E, Terzi RM, Kucharczyk N and Sofia RD (1985) The comparative potency of phenobarbital and five 1,3-propanediol dicarbamates for hepatic cytochrome P450 induction in rats. *Res. Commun. Path. Pharmac.*, **48**, 467–470.

Smart HL, Somerville KW, Williams J, Richens A and Langman MJC (1985) The effect of sucralfate upon phenytoin absorption in man. *Br. J. Clin. Pharmacol.*, **20**, 238–240.

Southern AL, Gordon GG, Tochimoto S *et al.* (1969) Effect of N-phenylbarbital on the metabolism of testosterone and cortisol in man. *J. Clin. Endocrinol.*, **29**, 251–286.

Spector R, Park GD, Johnson GG and Vesell ES (1988) Therapeutic drug monitoring. *Clin. Pharmacol. Therap.*, **43**, 345–353.

Stjernholm MR and Katz FH (1975) Effects of diphenylhydantoin, phenobarbital and diazepam on the metabolism of methylprednisolone and its sodium succinate. *J. Clin. Endocrinol. Metab.*, **41**, 887–893.

Stolarek I, Blacklaw J, Thompson GG and Brodie MJ (1994) Vigabatrin and lamotrigine in refractory epilepsy. *J. Neurol. Neurosurg. Psychiatry* (in press).

Swinyard EA, Woodhead JH, Franklin MR, Sofia RD and Kupferberg HJ (1987) The effect of chronic felbamate administration on anticonvulsant activity and hepatic drug-metabolising enzymes in mice and rats. *Epilepsia,* **28**, 295–300.

Tartara A, Galimberti CA, Manni R *et al.* (1993) The pharmacokinetics of oxcarbazepine and its active metabolite 10-hydroxycarbazepine in healthy subjects and in epileptic patients treated with phenobarbitone or valproic acid. *Br. J. Clin. Pharmacol.,* **36**, 366–368.

Thomson AH and Brodie MJ (1992) Pharmacokinetic optimisation of anticonvulsant therapy. *Clin. Pharmacokinet.,* **23**, 216–230.

Tomson T, Almqvist O, Nilsson BY, Svensson J-O and Bertilsson L (1990) Carbamazepine 10,11 epoxide in epilepsy, a pilot study. *Arch. Neurol.,* **47**, 888–892.

Vincent FM (1980) Phenothiazine-induced phenytoin intoxication. *Ann. Int. Med.,* **93**, 56–57.

Wagner ML, Leppik IE, Graves NM, Renne RP and Campbell JI (1990) Felbamate serum concentrations: effect of valproate, carbamazepine, phenytoin and phenobarbital. *Epilepsia,* **31**, 642.

Wagner ML, Graves NM, Leppik IE, Remmel RP, Ward DL and Schumaker RC (1991a) The effect of felbamate on valproate disposition. *Epilepsia,* **32**, 15.

Wagner ML, Graves NM, Marienau K, Holmes GB, Remmel RP and Leppik IE (1991b) Discontinuation of phenytoin and carbamazepine in patients receiving felbamate. *Epilepsia,* **32**, 398–406.

Warner T, Patsalos PN, Prevett M, Elyas AA and Duncan JS (1992) Lamotrigine-induced carbamazepine toxicity: an interaction with carbamazepine 10,11 epoxide. *Epilepsy Res.,* **11**, 147–150.

Wassner SJ, Pennisi AJ, Malėkzadeh MH and Fine RH (1976) The adverse effect of anticonvulsant therapy on renal allograft survival. *J. Paed.,* **88**, 134–137.

Werk EE, Choi Y, Sholiton L, Olinger C and Haque N (1969) Interference in the effect of dexamethasone by diphenylhydantoin. *N. Eng. J. Med.,* **281**, 32–34.

Werk EG, McGee J and Sholiton LJ (1964) Effect of diphenylhydantoin on cortisol metabolism in man. *J. Clin. Invest.,* **43**, 1824–1835.

Wolf P (1992) Lamotrigine: preliminary clinical observations on pharmacokinetics and interactions with traditional antiepileptic drugs. *J. Epilepsy,* **5**, 73–79.

Wong YY, Ludden TM and Bell R (1983) Effect of erythromycin on carbamazepine kinetics. *Clin. Pharmacol. Therap.,* **33**, 460–464.

Yuen AWC, Land G, Weatherby BC and Peck AW (1992) Sodium valproate acutely inhibits lamotrigine metabolism. *Br. J. Clin. Pharmacol.,* **33**, 511–513.

Zaccara G, Gangemi PF, Bendoni L, Menge GP, Schwabe S and Monza GC (1993) Influence of single and repeated doses of oxcarbazepine on the pharmacokinetic profile of felodipine. *Ther. Drug Monit.,* **15**, 39–42.

Zielinski JJ and Haidukewych D (1987) Dual effect of carbamazepine–phenytoin interaction. *Ther. Drug Monit.,* **9**, 21–23.

# 2

# Mechanisms of action of new anticonvulsant drugs

ROBERT L. MACDONALD AND KEVIN M. KELLY
*University of Michigan Medical Center, Ann Arbor, Michigan, USA*

## INTRODUCTION

A limited number of anticonvulsant drugs are currently available for use in the treatment of patients with epilepsy. Until recently, drugs were limited primarily to phenytoin, carbamazepine, barbiturates and primidone, benzodiazepines, valproic acid and ethosuximide. Recently, a number of additional compounds have become available. Five promising new anticonvulsants include gabapentin, felbamate, lamotrigine, oxcarbazepine and vigabatrin. Actions of these drugs at neurotransmitter receptors or ion channels may be responsible for their clinical effects. Three primary neurotransmitter receptor or ion channels are targeted by the currently used drugs and by some of the newly developed ones: gamma-aminobutyric acid A ($GABA_A$) receptor channels, voltage-dependent sodium channels and voltage-dependent low threshold (T-type) calcium channels. The interaction of the new anticonvulsants with specific neurotransmitter receptors or ion channels is the subject of this chapter.

## FELBAMATE

Felbamate, 2-phenyl-1,3-propanediol dicarbamate, is a dicarbamate that has a structure similar to meprobamate, an antianxiety agent (Figure 1). In experimental animals, felbamate was effective in blocking seizures induced by maximal electroshock, pentylenetetrazol and picrotoxin (Swinyard *et al.*, 1986). Felbamate inhibited bicuculline-induced seizures at high concentrations but

*New Anticonvulsants: Advances in the Treatment of Epilepsy.* Edited by M. R. Trimble
© 1994 John Wiley & Sons Ltd

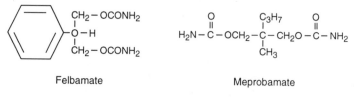

Felbamate                                    Meprobamate

**Figure 1.**   Structure of felbamate and meprobamate

was ineffective against strychnine-induced seizures (Sofia *et al.*, 1991). In sub-protective doses, felbamate enhanced the protective effects of diazepam against seizures induced by maximal electroshock, pentylenetetrazol and iso-niazid, but not bicuculline, suggesting that felbamate may have indirect effects on the $GABA_A$ receptor complex or be involved in other mechanisms of action (Gordon *et al.*, 1991). In clinical studies, felbamate has been effective in the treatment of partial seizures with and without secondary generalization in adults and partial and generalized seizures associated with the Lennox–Gastaut syndrome in children.

Felbamate has been tested for interaction with the $GABA_A$ receptor complex as a possible mechanism of its anticonvulsant activity. In rat brain cortical membranes, felbamate did not affect ligand binding to the GABA, benzodiazepine or picrotoxin binding sites of the $GABA_A$ receptor complex, and in radiolabelled chloride ion influx studies in cultured mouse spinal cord neurons, felbamate did not affect GABA-induced Cl⁻ influx (Ticku *et al.*, 1991). However, in cultural rat hippocampal neurons, felbamate produced an increase in GABA-evoked Cl⁻ currents which was not blocked by the benzodiazepine receptor antagonist flumazenil, suggesting that felbamate was active at the $GABA_A$ receptor complex but not as an agonist at the benzodiazepine recognition site (Rho *et al.*, 1993).

In other studies using mouse spinal cord neurons, felbamate reduced sustained repetitive firing of action potentials of voltage-dependent sodium channels ($IC_{50}$ of 67 μg/ml when compared with a control population of neurons of which 72% responded with sustained repetitive firing) (White *et al.*, 1992). It remains to be determined whether these results indicate a direct interaction of felbamate with voltage-dependent sodium channels.

Felbamate has also been tested for a possible effect on excitatory amino acid receptors. Felbamate inhibited seizures induced by N-methyl-D-aspartate (NMDA) and quisqualate in mice, but did not significantly inhibit MK-801 binding (Sofia *et al.*, 1991). Felbamate has been shown to inhibit the binding of [³H]5,7-dichlorokynurenic acid, a competitive antagonist, at the strychnine-insensitive glycine site of the NMDA receptor (McCabe *et al.*, 1993). It also reduced the ability of glycine to enhance NMDA-induced calcium currents in cerebellar granule cells measured by the fluorescent probe indo-1. In other studies, D-serine, a glycine site agonist, was administered intracerebroventricularly in audiogenic seizure-susceptible mice and produced a parallel right shift in felbamate's anticonvulsant dose–response curve (Harmsworth *et al.*, 1993). The results of these different studies suggest that felbamate has activity at the glycine site of the NMDA receptor that may be related to its anticonvulsant mechanism of action. However, studies in cultured rat hippocampal neurons showed that felbamate's inhibition of NMDA receptor currents could not be overcome by increasing the concentration of NMDA or glycine, suggesting that this drug's activity was more consistent with open channel block than with antagonism at the glycine site of the NMDA receptor (Rho *et al.*, 1993).

Further experiments are required to characterize more fully the potential anticonvulsant mechanisms of action of felbamate. These mechanisms of action may include enhancement of GABA$_A$ receptor-mediated inhibition, inhibition of high-frequency repetitive firing of sodium channels, and inhibition at the NMDA receptor ion channel complex. Diverse mechanisms of action of this drug may underlie its unique anticonvulsant profile and clinical effectiveness.

## GABAPENTIN

Gabapentin, 1-(aminomethyl)cyclohexaneacetic acid, is a cyclic GABA analogue (Figure 2) originally designed to mimic the steric conformation of GABA (Schmidt, 1989), to have high lipid solubility to penetrate the blood–brain barrier, and to be a centrally active GABA agonist with potential therapeutic value (Rogawski and Porter, 1990). Gabapentin has been shown to have anticonvulsant activity in a variety of animal seizure models (Bartoszyk *et al.*, 1986) and is effective in the treatment of human partial and generalized tonic–clonic seizures.

Early work with gabapentin suggested that it might act on GABAergic neurotransmitter systems since it protected mice from tonic extension in

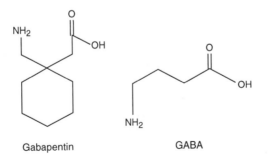

Gabapentin            GABA

**Figure 2.**   Structure of gabapentin and GABA

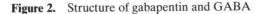

chemical convulsion models using inhibitors of GABA synthesis (3-mercaptopropionic acid, isonicotinic acid, semicarbazide) or antagonists acting at the $GABA_A$ receptor complex (bicuculline, picrotoxin) (Bartoszyk et al., 1983; Bartoszyk and Reimann, 1985). However, subsequent work has not clearly demonstrated a specific effect of gabapentin on GABAergic neuro-transmitter systems. Inhibition of monoamine release by gabapentin in elec-trically stimulated rabbit caudate nucleus (Reimann, 1983) and rat cortex (Schlicker et al., 1985) was not modified by GABA, baclofen or bicuculline, suggesting that gabapentin did not act at $GABA_A$ or $GABA_B$ receptors. Bind-ing experiments in rat brain and spinal cord have shown that this drug has no significant affinity for the $GABA_A$ or $GABA_B$ binding sites measured by $^3H$-muscimol and $^3H$-baclofen displacement, respectively. Gabapentin did not sig-nificantly inhibit the binding of $^3H$-diazepam, had only a weak inhibitory effect on the GABA degrading enzyme GABA aminotransferase, did not elevate GABA content in nerve terminals, and did not affect the GABA uptake system (Bartoszyk et al., 1986). However, gabapentin has been shown to increase GABA turnover in several regions of rat brain (Loscher et al., 1991).

Recent work has shown that gabapentin binds to a novel high-affinity site in the central nervous system (Hill et al., 1993; Suman-Chauhan et al., 1993; Chapter 5) and was potently displaced by the anticonvulsant 3-isobutyl GABA (Taylor et al., 1993), but the identity of this binding site remains uncertain. Additionally, gabapentin has been shown to be a substrate for a saturable L-amino acid transport system in rat gut tissues (Stewart et al., 1994), and appeared to be concentrated from brain interstitial fluid into brain tissue by an active process (Welty et al., 1994). The results of these studies raise the possibility of a specific binding site of gabapentin for active transport across neuronal membranes. This hypothesis remains to be tested.

In electrophysiological studies, gabapentin did not affect depolarizations elicited by iontophoretic application of GABA on cultured mouse spinal cord neurons (Taylor et al., 1988; Rock et al., 1993). Additionally, this drug appeared to act by GABA receptor-independent mechanisms in studies with rat hippocampal slices (Haas and Wieser, 1986) and the feline trigeminal nucleus (Kondo et al., 1991). Gabapentin has been shown to decrease inhibi-tion evoked by paired-pulse orthodromic stimulation of pyramidal neurons in the hippocampal slice preparation (Dooley et al., 1985; Taylor et al., 1988); however, the specific effect of the drug in this paradigm is not known.

Gabapentin protected mice from convulsions caused by strychnine, a glycine receptor antagonist, but was unable to displace $^3H$-strychnine in bind-ing studies at the highest concentrations tested (Bartoszyk et al., 1986). Elec-trophysiological studies showed no effect of the drug on the response of spinal cord neurons to iontophoretically applied glycine (Rock et al., 1993).

Gabapentin has been tested in animal seizure models where seizures are induced by administration of excitatory amino acids. It prolonged the onset latency of clonic convulsions, tonic extension and death in mice following intraperitoneal injections of NMDA, but not of kainic acid or quinolinic acid. The drug did not have a clear effect on convulsions when these compounds or glutamate were injected into the lateral ventricle of rats (Bartoszyk, 1983). Intraperitoneal injections in mice of gabapentin or the NMDA receptor competitive antagonist 3-((±)-2-carboxypiperazin-4-yl)-propyl-1-phosphonic acid (CPP) antagonized tonic seizures. The effect of gabapentin, but not CPP, was dose-dependently antagonized by the administration of serine, an agonist at the glycine receptor on the NMDA receptor complex, suggesting an involvement of the strychnine-insensitive glycine site of the NMDA receptor in the anticonvulsant activity of gabapentin (Oles et al., 1990).

In unpublished studies, gabapentin reportedly antagonized NMDA-induced (but not kainate-induced) depolarizations in thalamic and hippocampal slice preparations, and antagonized NMDA-induced currents in the presence of glycine in cultured striatal neurons, an effect that was reversed by the addition of serine or increased glycine (Chadwick, 1992). Other studies did not show a significant effect of gabapentin on neuronal responses to iontophoretic application of glutamate or on membrane depolarizations and single channel currents evoked by NMDA with or without coapplication of glycine (Rock et al., 1993). These results, in part, are similar to the findings of others where gabapentin had no effect on spinal cord neuron depolarizations elicited by iontophoretically applied glutamate (Taylor et al., 1988) or pressure-ejected NMDA (Wamil et al., 1991). Additionally, in extracellular recordings from rat hippocampal slice preparations, gabapentin had no effect on long-term potentiation, making it unlike NMDA receptor antagonists (Taylor et al., 1988).

Gabapentin had no effect on sustained repetitive firing of action potentials in mouse spinal cord neurons (Taylor et al., 1988; Rock et al., 1993). In other experiments using the same neuronal preparation, prolonged times of exposure (12–48 hours) and/or application of gabapentin resulted in a voltage-dependent and frequency-dependent limitation of sustained repetitive firing of sodium action potentials at therapeutically relevant concentrations (Wamil et al., 1994). However, gabapentin had no effect on rat brain type IIA sodium channel $\alpha$ subunit currents expressed in Chinese hamster ovary cells following 24-hour bath application of gabapentin, or when the drug was delivered by blunt pipette or the recording electrode (Taylor, 1993). The results of these different studies suggest that the anticonvulsant activity of gabapentin is not due to a direct interaction with voltage-dependent sodium channels limiting sustained repetitive firing of action potentials.

Although gabapentin is most effective in the treatment of human partial and generalized tonic–clonic seizures, its effect on absence seizures has been studied in both animal models of absence seizures and as add-on therapy in patients with epilepsy who are drug-resistant. In animal studies using pentylenetetrazol-induced clonic seizures, gabapentin protected mice from clonic convulsions in both the subcutaneous metrazol test and the intravenous threshold test (Bartoszyk et al., 1986). However, in a rat genetic model of absence epilepsy, this drug increased electroencephalographic spike and wave bursts in a dose-dependent manner (Foot and Wallace, 1991). In human studies, gabapentin reduced absence seizures by more than 50% in half of the patients in one study (Bauer et al., 1989), and in another study, the drug reduced absence seizures and generalized spike and wave complexes in patients undergoing 24-hour electroencephalogram monitoring (Rowan et al., 1989). In studies of mouse spinal cord neurons, gabapentin blocked responses to Bay K 8644, an agonist at the dihydropyridine binding site of the L-type calcium channel (Wamil et al., 1991). In other electrophysiological studies, however, this drug did not significantly affect any calcium channel current subtype (T, N or L), suggesting that its basic mechanism of action was not on voltage-dependent calcium channels (Rock et al., 1993).

In summary, the results of several studies have not demonstrated a major effect of gabapentin on ligand-gated or voltage-gated channels. Further work on the high-affinity binding site of gabapentin and the possibility of active transport of the drug across neuronal membranes should contribute significantly to understanding its mechanism of action.

## LAMOTRIGINE

Lamotrigine, 3,5-diamino-6-(2,3-dichlorophenyl)-1,2,4-triazine (Figure 3), is a phenyltriazine with weak antifolate activity. The drug was developed following observations that use of phenobarbitone, primidone and phenytoin resulted in reduced folate levels and that folates could induce seizures in experimental animals (Reynolds et al., 1966). It was proposed that antifolate activity may be related to anticonvulsant activity; however, this has not been demonstrated by structure–activity studies (Rogawski and Porter, 1990). Lamotrigine has anticonvulsant activity in several animal seizure models, including hind-limb extension in maximal electroshock and maximal pentylenetetrazol seizures in rodents (Miller et al., 1986). It has been effective as add-on therapy in the treatment of human partial and generalized tonic–clonic seizures.

The action of lamotrigine on the release of endogenous amino acids from rat cerebral cortex slices in vitro has been studied. Lamotrigine potently inhibited release of glutamate and aspartate evoked by the sodium channel activator veratrine and was much less effective in the inhibition of release of acetylcholine or GABA. At high concentrations, it had no effect on spontaneous or potassium-evoked amino acid release. These studies suggested that this drug acted at voltage-dependent sodium channels resulting in decreased

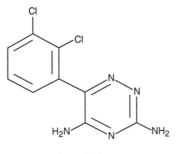

Lamotrigine

**Figure 3.** Structure of lamotrigine

presynaptic release of glutamate (Leach *et al.*, 1986). In radioligand studies, the binding of $^3$H-batrachotoxinin A 20-α-benzoate, a neurotoxin that binds to receptor sites 2 on voltage-dependent sodium channels, was inhibited by lamotrigine in rat brain synaptosomes (Cheung *et al.*, 1992). Several electrophysiological studies have tested the effects of lamotrigine on voltage-dependent sodium channels. The drug blocked sustained repetitive firing in cultured mouse spinal cord neurons in a dose-dependent manner at concentrations therapeutic in the treatment of human seizures (Cheung *et al.*, 1992). In cultured rat cortical neurons, lamotrigine reduced burst firing induced by glutamate or potassium, but not unitary sodium action potentials evoked at low frequencies (Lees and Leach, 1993). In cultured hippocampal neurons, this drug reduced sodium currents in a voltage-dependent manner, and at depolarized potentials showed a small frequency-dependent inhibition (Mutoh and Dichter, 1993). Lamotrigine increased steady state inactivation of rat brain type IIA sodium channel α subunit currents expressed in Chinese hamster ovary cells (Taylor, 1993) and produced both tonic and frequency-dependent inhibition of voltage-dependent sodium channels in clonal N4TG1 mouse neuroblastoma cells, but had no effect on cationic currents induced by stimulation of glutamatergic receptors in embryonic rat hippocampal neurons (Wang *et al.*, 1993).

In cultured rat cortical neurons, lamotrigine at high concentrations was able to inhibit peak high threshold calcium currents and appeared to shift the threshold for inward currents to more depolarized potentials (Lees and Leach, 1993). In clonal rat pituitary GH3 cells, lamotrigine at the same concentration did not inhibit high threshold calcium currents, caused only slight inhibition of low threshold calcium currents, reduced rapidly inactivating voltage-dependent potassium currents, and had no significant effect on calcium-activated potassium currents (Lang and Wang, 1991). In cultured rat cortical neurons, lamotrigine did not appear to mimic the effect of diazepam when tested on GABA-evoked chloride currents (Lees and Leach, 1993).

These results suggest that the anticonvulsant effect of lamotrigine is due to a specific interaction at the voltage-dependent sodium channel that results in voltage-dependent and frequency-dependent inhibition of the channel. These results are similar to those found for phenytoin and carbamazepine. It remains to be determined whether this action results in a significant preferential decreased release of presynaptic glutamate.

## OXCARBAZEPINE

Oxcarbazepine, 10,11-dihydro-10-oxocarbamazepine, is a derivative of the dibenzazepine series and is structurally very similar to carbamazepine (Figure 4). The drug differs from carbamazepine by a keto substitution at the 10,11 position of the dibenzazepine nucleus. The keto substitution causes a different biotransformation and greater tolerability in humans compared with carbamazepine. Oxcarbazepine is rapidly and nearly completely metabolized to 10,11-dihydro-10-hydroxycarbamazepine (GP 47779; HCBZ), the active metabolite which is responsible for the anticonvulsant activity of the drug

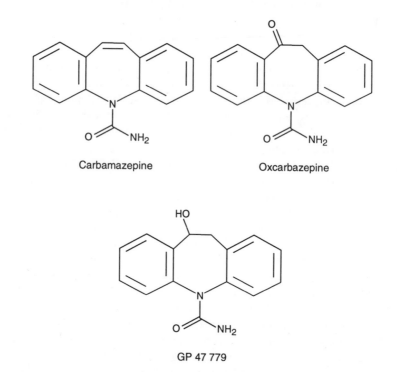

Carbamazepine             Oxcarbazepine

GP 47 779

**Figure 4.**  Structure of carbamazepine, oxycarbazepine and GB 47779

(Jensen *et al.*, 1991). HCBZ is a racemate with both enantiomers having approximately equal anticonvulsant activity (Schmutz *et al.*, 1993). Metabolism of oxcarbazepine does not result in the formation of 10,11-epoxycarbamazepine.

Oxcarbazepine and HCBZ are effective in inhibiting hind-limb extension in rats and mice elicited by maximal electroshock, but are approximately two to three times less effective against pentylenetetrazol-induced seizures in mice (Baltzer and Schmutz, 1978). In studies using rats at different developmental ages, oxcarbazepine, HCBZ and carbamazepine dose-dependently reduced the tonic phase of generalized seizures induced by pentylenetetrazol and appeared to have identical anticonvulsant profiles in this model (Kubova and Mares, 1993). Oxcarbazepine and HCBZ have relatively poor anticonvulsant efficacy against seizures induced by picrotoxin and strychnine in mice (Baltzer and Schmutz, 1978). Oxcarbazepine was able to completely suppress seizures in rhesus monkeys in a chronic aluminium foci model of partial seizures. At comparable doses, HCBZ was less effective in suppressing seizures in this model (Jensen *et al.*, 1991). Oxcarbazepine is effective in the treatment of human generalized tonic–clonic seizures and partial seizures with and without secondary generalization (Dam and Jensen, 1989).

In electrophysiological studies of rat hippocampal slices, oxcarbazepine and HCBZ enantiomers dose-dependently decreased epileptic-like discharges induced by penicillin. Additionally, the ability of these drugs to suppress discharges was decreased by 4-aminopyridine, a potassium channel blocker (Schmutz *et al.*, 1993). Because oxcarbazepine and HCBZ are similar to carbamazepine in both structure and clinical efficacy, it is tempting to speculate that their mechanism of action may be similar to that of carbamazepine, namely inhibition of sustained high-frequency repetitive firing of voltage-dependent sodium action potentials. However, this has not been demonstrated by electrophysiological testing, and the mechanism of action of oxcarbazepine remains unknown.

## VIGABATRIN

Vigabatrin (γ-vinyl GABA), 4-amino-hex-5-enoic acid, is a synthetic derivative and structural analogue of GABA (Figure 5). Vigabatrin was developed to be an enzyme-activated, irreversible inhibitor of GABA transaminase (GABA-T), the primary presynaptic degradative enzyme of GABA. Vigabatrin's selective inhibition of GABA-T was intended to have potential therapeutic value by increasing GABA levels in the brain and thereby enhance GABAergic transmission. The drug is a racemic mixture of S(+) and R(−) enantiomers. The S(+) enantiomer potently inhibits GABA-T whereas the R(−) enantiomer has minimal activity (Larsson *et al.*, 1986). The

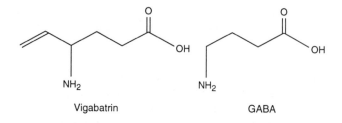

Vigabatrin GABA

**Figure 5.** Structure of vigabatrin and GABA

molecular mechanism of action of vigabatrin's inhibition of GABA-T has been proposed by Lippert et al. (1977). The drug is accepted as a substrate of GABA-T by forming a Schiff base with pyridoxal phosphate in the active site of the enzyme which abstracts a proton from the Schiff base. The resulting charge stabilization by the pyridine ring induces the aldimine to ketimine tautomerism that occurs in the normal transamination process. The reactive unsaturated ketimine forms a stable bond with a nucleophilic residue of GABA-T's active site, resulting in irreversible inhibition of the enzyme and eliminating its ability to transaminate new substrate.

Numerous animal studies have described the effects of vigabatrin's inhibition of GABA-T. Vigabatrin inhibited mouse whole brain GABA-T activity and increased whole brain GABA concentrations (Jung et al., 1977; Schechter et al., 1977). These actions were seen in all brain areas assayed and were quantitatively different, corresponding to the relative regional distribution of GABAergic neurons (Chapman et al., 1982).

In rat cortex, vigabatrin markedly increased the synaptosomal GABA pool compared with non-synaptosomal GABA (Sarhan and Seiler, 1979), suggesting a greater effect of the drug on neuronal GABA-T rather than on glial GABA-T. This effect is consistent with the finding that neurons have a high-affinity GABA uptake system, whereas astrocytes have a low-affinity system (Schousboe et al., 1986).

In human studies, vigabatrin dose-dependently increased cerebrospinal fluid levels of free and total GABA (Grove et al., 1981; Schechter et al., 1984; Ben-Menachem, 1989), but did not significantly affect other neurotransmitter systems (Schechter et al., 1984; Riekkinen et al., 1989). In recent studies with healthy subjects, nuclear magnetic resonance spectroscopy showed that occipital lobe GABA concentrations were elevated after vigabatrin was given (Petroff et al., 1993).

Vigabatrin has been shown to be an effective anticonvulsant in a variety of animal models of epilepsy. In studies with rodents, it inhibited strychnine-induced and audiogenic seizures (Schechter et al., 1979). Other studies showed that only the active S(+) enantiomer of vigabatrin was effective in inhibiting audiogenic seizures in mice (Meldrum and Murugaiah, 1983). Vigabatrin inhibited epileptic responses in photosensitive baboons (Meldrum and Horton, 1978), and inhibited the development of kindling (Shin et al., 1986; Loscher et al., 1987) as well as fully developed generalized seizures in the amygdala-kindled rat (Kalichman et al., 1982). It was less effective in inhibiting seizures caused by bicuculline and picrotoxin (Schechter and Tranier, 1977). Vigabatrin has been effective in the treatment of human partial seizures with or without secondary generalization.

In summary, vigabatrin is a selective irreversible inhibitor of GABA-T, the main degradative enzyme of GABA. Inhibition of GABA-T produces greater available pools of presynaptic GABA for release in central nervous system synapses. Increased activity of GABA at postsynaptic GABA receptors can cause increased inhibition of neurons important in controlling the abnormal electrical activity of seizures. These actions probably account for the clinical anticonvulsant effects of vigabatrin.

## CONCLUSION

The currently used anticonvulsant drugs appear to have only three major mechanisms of action (Table 1). Drugs that are effective against generalized tonic–clonic and partial seizures appear to reduce sustained high-frequency repetitive firing of action potentials by delaying recovery of sodium channels from activation. Drugs that are effective against generalized absence seizures appear to reduce low threshold (T-type) calcium currents. Finally, drugs that are effective against myoclonic seizures generally enhance $GABA_A$ receptor inhibition. While the currently available anticonvulsants have been shown to be effective, there are clearly a number of patients, especially those with complex partial seizures, whose seizures are refractory to them. The new drugs have shown considerable promise in clinical trials and may be of significant help in managing some refractory patients. While the mechanisms of action of these drugs are not fully established (Table 2), it is likely that additional new compounds that are under development will have actions on new neurotransmitter receptor or ion channels. For example, considerable effort has been directed toward developing agents that are antagonists of excitatory amino acid transmission. Hopefully, new anticonvulsants which act on different neurotransmitter receptors or ion channels will result in improved control of seizures in patients refractory to currently available anticonvulsant therapy.

Approaches to the investigation of the mechanisms of action of anticonvulsants to date have been fairly descriptive. With the application of new molecular biological techniques to the study of central nervous system function and the cloning of cDNAs for specific neurotransmitter receptors and ion channels that are targets of anticonvulsant therapy, it may be possible to study the

**Table 1.**   Anticonvulsant drug actions

|  | Sodium channels | GABA$_A$ receptors | T-type calcium channels |
|---|---|---|---|
| Carbamazepine | ++ | – | – |
| Phenytoin | ++ | – | – |
| Primidone | + | – | ? |
| Valproic acid | ++ | ?/+ | ?/+ |
| Barbiturates | + | + | – |
| Benzodiazepines | + | ++ | – |
| Ethosuximide | – | – | ++ |

**Table 2.**   New anticonvulsant drug actions

|  | Sodium channels | GABA$_A$ receptors | T-type calcium channels | NMDA receptor |
|---|---|---|---|---|
| Felbamate | +/? | +/? | ? | +/? |
| Gabapentin | +/? | – | – | – |
| Lamotrigine | ++ | –/? | –/? | ? |
| Oxcarbazepine | +/? | ? | ? | ? |
| Vigabatrin | ? | + | ? | ? |

interaction of these drugs with their molecular targets in more detail. Insights gained from these studies may assist in the design of improved anticonvulsants which may act on the same receptors or ion channels but have more specific and selective actions.

## REFERENCES

Baltzer V and Schmutz M (1978) Experimental anticonvulsive properties of GP 47 680 and of GP 47 779, its main human metabolite; compounds related to carbamazepine. In: *Advances in Epileptology, 1977* (eds H Meinardi and J Rowan), pp. 295–299. Swets & Zeitlinger, Amsterdam.

Bartoszyk GD (1983) Gabapentin and convulsions provoked by excitatory amino acids. *Naunyn-Schmiedeberg's Arch. Pharmacol.*, **324**, R24.

Bartoszyk GC and Reimann W (1985) Preclinical characterization of the anticonvulsant gabapentin. *16th Epilepsy International Congress*, Hamburg.

Bartoszyk GD, Fritschi E, Herrmann M and Satzinger G (1983) Indications for an involvement of the GABA-system in the mechanism of action of gabapentin. *Naunyn-Schmiedeberg's Arch. Pharmacol.*, **322**, R94.

Bartoszyk GD, Meyerson N, Reimann W, Satzinger G and von Hodenberg A (1986) Gabapentin. In: *Current Problems in Epilepsy: New Anticonvulsant Drugs* (eds BS Meldrum and RJ Porter), pp. 147–164. John Libbey, London.

Bauer G, Bechinger D, Castell M *et al.* (1989) Gabapentin in the treatment of drug-resistant epileptic patients. *Adv. Epileptol.*, **17**, 219–221.

Ben-Menachem E (1989) Pharmacokinetic effects of vigabatrin on cerebrospinal fluid amino acids in humans. *Epilepsia,* **30** (suppl. 3), S12–14.

Chadwick D (1992) Gabapentin. In: *Recent Advances in Epilepsy* (eds TA Pedley and BS Meldrum), pp. 211–221. Churchill Livingstone, New York.

Chapman AG, Riley K, Evans MC and Meldrum BS (1982) Acute effects of sodium valproate and γ-vinyl GABA on regional amino acid metabolism in the rat brain: incorporation of 2-[$^{14}$C]glucose into amino acids. *Neurochem. Res.,* **7**, 1089–1105.

Cheung H, Kamp D and Harris E (1992) An in vitro investigation of the action of lamotrigine on neuronal voltage-activated sodium channels. *Epilepsy Res.,* **13**(2), 107–112.

Dam M and Jensen PK (1989) Potential antiepileptic drugs: oxcarbazepine. In: *Antiepileptic Drugs,* 3rd edn (eds RH Levy, FE Driefuss, RH Mattson, BS Meldrum and JK Penry), pp. 913–924. Raven Press, New York.

Dooley DJ, Bartoszyk GD, Rock DM and Satzinger G (1985) Preclinical characterization of the anticonvulsant gabapentin. *16th Epilepsy International Congress,* Hamburg.

Foot M and Wallace J (1991) Gabapentin. In: *New Antiepileptic Drugs (Epilepsy Res.,* suppl. 3) (eds F Pisani, E Perucca, G Avazini and A Richens), pp. 109–114. Elsevier, Amsterdam.

Gordon R, Gels M, Diamantis W and Sofia RD (1991) Interaction of felbamate and diazepam against maximum electroshock seizures and chemoconvulsants in mice. *Pharmacol. Biochem. Behav.,* **40**, 109–113.

Grove J, Schechter PJ, Tell G *et al.* (1981) Increased gamma-aminobutyric acid (GABA), homocarnosine and β-alanine in cerebrospinal fluid of patients treated with gamma-vinyl GABA (4-amino-hex-5-enoic acid). *Life Sci.,* **28**, 2431–2439.

Haas HL and Wieser HG (1986) Gabapentin: action on hippocampal slices of the rat and effects in human epileptics. *Northern European Epilepsy Meeting,* York.

Harmsworth WL, Wolf HH, Swinyard EA and White HS (1993) Felbamate modulates glycine receptor function. *Epilepsia,* **34** (suppl. 2), 92–93.

Hill, DR, Suman-Chauhan N and Woodruff GN (1993) Localisation of [$^3$H]gabapentin to a novel site in rat brain: autoradiographic studies. *Eur. J. Pharmacol. Mol. Pharmacol.,* **244**, 303–309.

Jensen PK, Gram L and Schmutz M (1991) Oxcarbazepine. In: *New Antiepileptic Drugs (Epilepsy Res.,* suppl. 3) (eds F Pisani, E Perucca, G Avanzini and A Richens), pp. 135–140. Elsevier, Amsterdam.

Jung MJ, Lippert B, Metcalf B, Bohlen P and Schechter PJ (1977) γ-Vinyl GABA (4-amino-hex-5-enoic acid), a new irreversible inhibitor of GABA-T: effects on brain GABA metabolism in mice. *J. Neurochem.,* **29**, 797–802.

Kalichman MW, Burnham WM and Livingstone KE (1982) Pharmacological investigation of gamma-aminobutyric acid (GABA) and fully developed generalized seizures in the amygdala-kindled rat. *Neuropharmacology,* **21**, 127–131.

Kondo T, Fromm GH and Schmidt B (1991) Comparison of gabapentin with other antiepileptic and GABAergic drugs. *Epilepsy Res.,* **8**, 226–231.

Kubova H and Mares P (1993) Anticonvulsant action of oxcarbazepine, hydroxycarbamazepine, and carbamazepine against metrazol-induced motor seizures in developing rats. *Epilepsia,* **34**, 188–192.

Lang DG and Wang CM (1991) Lamotrigine and phenytoin interactions on ionic currents present in N4TG1 and GH3 clonal cells. *Soc. Neurosci. Abs.,* **17**, 1256.

Larsson OM, Gram L, Schousboe I and Schousboe A (1986) Differential effect of gamma-vinyl GABA and valproate on GABA-transaminase from cultured neurones and astrocytes. *Neuropharmacology,* **25**, 617–625.

Leach MJ, Marden CM and Miller AA (1986) Pharmacological studies on lamotrigine, a novel potential antiepileptic drug: II. Neurochemical studies on the mechanism of action. *Epilepsia,* **27** (5), 490–497.

Lees G and Leach MJ (1993) Studies on the mechanism of action of the novel anticonvulsant lamotrigine (Lamictal) using primary neurological cultures from rat cortex. *Brain Res.,* **612**, 190–199.

Lippert B, Metcalf BW, Jung MJ and Casara P (1977) 4-Amino-hex-5-enoic acid, a selective catalytic inhibitor of 4-aminobutyric-acid aminotransferase in mammalian brain. *Eur. J. Biochem.,* **74**, 441–445.

Loscher W, Czuczwar SJ, Jackel R and Schwarz M (1987) Effect of microinjections of gamma-vinyl GABA or isoniazid into substantia nigra on the development of amygdala kindling in rats. *Exp. Neurol.,* **95**, 622–638.

Loscher W, Honack D and Taylor CP (1991) Gabapentin increases aminooxyacetic acid-induced GABA accumulation in several regions of rat brain. *Neurosci. Lett.,* **128**, 150–154.

McCabe RT, Wasterlain CG, Kucharczyk N, Sofia RD and Vogel JR (1993) Evidence of anticonvulsant and neuroprotectant action of felbamate mediated by strychnine-insensitive glycine receptors. *J. Pharmacol. Exp. Ther.,* **264** (3), 248–252.

Meldrum BS and Horton R (1978) Blockade of epileptic responses in photosensitive baboon *Papio papio* by two irreversible inhibitors of GABA-transaminase, gamma-acetylenic GABA (4-amino-hex-5-ynoic acid) and gamma-vinyl GABA (4-amino-hex-5-enoic acid). *Psychopharmacologia,* **59**, 47–50.

Meldrum BS and Murugaiah K (1983) Anticonvulsant action in mice with sound-induced seizures of the optical isomers of gamma vinyl GABA. *Eur. J. Pharmacol.,* **89**, 149–152.

Miller AA, Wheatley P, Sawyer DA, Baxter MG and Roth B (1986) Pharmacological studies on lamotrigine, a novel potential antiepileptic drug: I. Anticonvulsant profile in mice and rats. *Epilepsia,* **27** (5), 483–489.

Mutoh K and Dichter MA (1993) Lamotrigine blocks voltage-dependent Na currents in a voltage-dependent manner with a small use-dependent component. *Epilepsia,* **34** (suppl. 6), 87.

Oles RJ, Singh L, Hughes J and Woodruff GN (1990) The anticonvulsant action of gabapentin involves the glycine/NMDA receptor. *Soc. Neurosci. Abs.,* **16**, 783.

Petroff OAC, Rothman DL, Behar KL and Mattson RH (1993) Effect of vigabatrin on GABA levels in human brain measured in vivo with [$^1$H] NMR spectroscopy. *Epilepsia,* **34** (suppl. 6), 68.

Reimann W (1983) Inhibition of GABA, baclofen, and gabapentin of dopamine release from rabbit caudate nucleus: are there common or different sites of action? *Eur. J. Pharmacol.,* **94**, 341–344.

Reynolds EH, Milner G, Matthews DM and Chanarin I (1966) Anticonvulsant therapy, megaloblastic haemopoiesis and folic acid metabolism. *Quart. J. Med.,* **35**, 521–537.

Rho JM, Donevan SD and Rogawski MA (1994) Mechanism of action of the anticonvulsant felbamate: opposing effects on *N*-methy-D-aspartate and γ-aminobutyric acid$_A$ receptors. *Annals of Neurology,* **35**, 229–234.

Riekkinen PJ, Pitkanen A, Ylinen A, Sivenius J and Halonen T (1989) Specificity of vigabatrin for the GABAergic system in human epilepsy. *Epilepsia,* **30** (suppl. 3), S18–22.

Rock DM, Kelly KM and Macdonald RL (1993) Gabapentin actions on ligand- and voltage-gated responses in cultured rodent neurons. *Epilepsy Res.,* **16**, 89–98.

Rogawski MA and Porter RJ (1990) Antiepileptic drugs: pharmacological mechanisms and clinical efficacy with consideration of promising developmental stage compounds. *Pharmacol. Rev.*, **42**, 223–286.

Rowan AJ, Schear MJ, Wiener JA and Luciano D (1989) Intensive monitoring and pharmacokinetic studies of gabapentin in patients with generalized spike-wave discharges. *Epilepsia*, **30**, 30.

Sarhan S and Seiler N (1979) Metabolic inhibitors and subcellular distribution of GABA. *J. Neurosci. Res.*, **4**, 399–421.

Schechter PJ and Tranier Y (1977) Effects of elevated brain GABA concentrations on the action of bicuculline and picrotoxin in mice. *Psychopharmacology*, **54**, 145–148.

Schechter PJ, Trainier Y, Jung MJ and Bohlen P (1977) Audiogenic seizure protection by elevated brain GABA concentration in mice: effects of γ-acetylenic GABA and γ-vinyl GABA, two irreversible GABA-T inhibitors. *Eur. J. Pharmacol.*, **45**, 319–328.

Schechter PJ, Tranier Y and Grove J (1979) Attempts to correlate alterations in brain GABA metabolism by GABA-T inhibitors with their anticonvulsant effect. In: *GABA-Biochemistry and CNS Function* (eds P Mandel and FV DeFeudis), pp. 43–57. Plenum Press, New York.

Schechter PJ, Hanke NFJ, Grove J, Huebert N and Sjoerdsma A (1984) Biochemical and clinical effects of gamma-vinyl GABA in patients with epilepsy. *Neurology*, **34**, 182–186.

Schlicker E, Reimann W and Gothert M (1985) Gabapentin decreases monoamine release without affecting acetylcholine release in the brain. *Arzneim.-Forsch./Drug Res.*, **35**, 1347–1349.

Schmidt D (1989) Potential antiepileptic drugs: gabapentin. In: *Antiepileptic Drugs*, 3rd edn (eds RH Levy, FE Driefuss, RH Mattson, BS Meldrum and JK Penry, pp. 925–935. Raven Press, New York.

Schmutz M, Ferret T, Heckendorn R, Jeker A, Portet C and Olpe HR (1993) GP 47779, the main human metabolite of oxcarbazepine (Trileptal), and both enantiomers have equal anticonvulsant activity. *Epilepsia*, **34** (suppl. 2), 122.

Schousboe A, Larsson OM and Seiler N (1986) Stereoselective uptake of the GABA-transaminase inhibitors gamma-vinyl GABA and gamma-acetylenic GABA into neurons and astrocytes. *Neurochem. Res.*, **11**, 1497–1505.

Shin C, Rigsbee LC and McNamara JO (1986) Anti-seizure and anti-epileptogenic effect of gamma-vinyl gamma-aminobutyric acid in amygdaloid kindling. *Brain Res.*, **398**, 370–374.

Sofia RD, Kramer L, Perhach JL and Rosenberg A (1991) Felbamate. In: *New Antiepileptic Drugs (Epilepsy Res.,* suppl. 3) (eds F Pisani, E Perucca, G Avanzini and A Richens), pp. 103–108. Elsevier, Amsterdam.

Stewart BH, Kugler AR, Thompson PR and Bockbrader HN (1993) A saturable transport mechanism in the intestinal absorption of gabapentin is the underlying cause of the lack of proportionality between increasing dose and drug levels in plasma. *Pharmaceut. Res.*, **10**, 276–81.

Suman-Chauhan N, Webdale L, Hill DR and Woodruff GN (1993) Characterisation of [3H]gabapentin binding to a novel site in rat brain: homogenate binding studies. *Eur. J. Pharmacol.*, **244**, 293–301.

Swinyard EA, Sofia RD and Kupferberg HJ (1986) Comparative anticonvulsant activity and neurotoxicity of felbamate and four protype antiepileptic drugs in mice and rats. *Epilepsia*, **27**, 27–34.

Taylor CP (1993) The anticonvulsant lamotrigine blocks sodium currents from cloned alpha-subunits of rat brain Na⁺ channels in a voltage-dependent manner but gabapentin does not. *Soc. Neurosci. Abs.,* **19**, 1631.

Taylor CP, Rock DM, Weinkauf RJ and Ganong AH (1988) In vitro and in vivo electrophysiological effects of the anticonvulsant gabapentin. *Soc. Neurosci. Abs.,* **14**, 866.

Taylor CP, Vartanian MG, Yuen PW and Bigge C (1993) Potent and stereospecific anticonvulsant activity of 3-isobutyl GABA relates to in vitro binding at a novel site labeled by tritiated gabapentin. *Epilepsy Res.,* **14**, 11–15.

Ticku MK, Kamatchi GL and Sofia RD (1991) Effect of anticonvulsant felbamate on GABAA receptor system. *Epilepsia,* **32** (3), 389–391.

Wang CM, Lang DG and Cooper BR (1993) Lamotrigine effects on ion channels in cultured neuronal cells. *Epilepsia,* **34** (suppl. 6), 117–118.

Wamil AW and McLean MJ (1994) Limitation by gabapentin of high frequency action potential firing by mouse central neurons in cell culture. *Epilepsy Res.,* **17**, 1-10.

Wamil AW, McLean MJ and Taylor CP (1991) Multiple cellular actions of gabapentin. *Neurology,* **41** (suppl. 1), 140.

Welty DF, Schielke GP, Vartanian MG and Taylor CP (1993) Gabapentin anticonvulsant action in rats: disequilibrium with peak drug concentrations in plasma and brain microdialysate. *Epilepsy Res.,* **16**, 175–181.

White HS, Wolf HH, Swinyard EA, Skeen GA and Sofia RD (1992) A neuropharmacological evaluation of felbamate as a novel anticonvulsant. *Epilepsia,* **33**, 564–572.

# 3

# Clobazam

MICHAEL R. TRIMBLE
*National Hospital for Neurology and Neurosurgery, London, UK*

## INTRODUCTION

Clobazam is intermediate between the older anticonvulsants and the newer ones. Thus, although some of the earliest clinical trials were reported in the late 1970s, its introduction into a number of countries was delayed. For example, it was licensed in Canada in 1991, some time after vigabatrin was introduced into the UK.

As a benzodiazepine, clobazam would be predicted to have anticonvulsant properties. However, generally benzodiazepines have not been found satisfactory for the oral management of seizures, there being a few notable exceptions. Table 1 gives a list of benzodiazepines that have been used orally in epilepsy; the majority of them are 1,4-benzodiazepines. Clobazam is a 1,5-benzodiazepine, the nitrogen on the heterocyclic ring being shifted by one position. This appears to confer on clobazam a more powerful anticonvulsant action, with less sedative and muscle relaxant properties, compared with the 1,4-benzodiazepines. Its structure is shown in Figure 1.

**Table 1.** Benzodiazepines that have been investigated in clinical studies for oral use

| |
| --- |
| Chlordiazepoxide |
| Clobazam |
| Clonazepam |
| Clorazepate |
| Diazepam |
| Lorazepam |
| Nitrazepam |
| Oxazepam |

*New Anticonvulsants: Advances in the Treatment of Epilepsy.* Edited by M. R. Trimble
© 1994 John Wiley & Sons Ltd

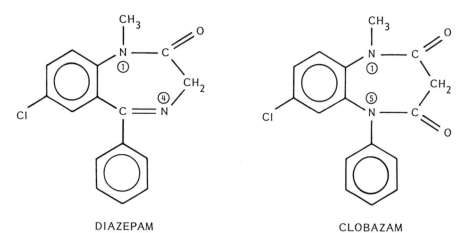

DIAZEPAM                          CLOBAZAM

**Figure 1.**   Structures of 1,4-benzodiazepine (left) and 1,5-benzodiazepine (right)

## PHARMACOLOGY

In human studies it has been shown that at least 87% of an oral dose of clobazam is absorbed, and, after single doses, clobazam reaches peak levels one to four hours later. It has a mean half-life of 18 hours (range 10 hours to 30 hours). After steady state has been reached, the levels of the main metabolite N-desmethylclobazam are about eight times higher than those of the parent compound, and its half-life is markedly longer than that of clobazam — 35–133 hours. This metabolite also possesses powerful anticonvulsant properties.

There is a linear correlation between clobazam dose and plasma levels of both the parent drug and its metabolite in healthy subjects (Rupp et al., 1979) and in patients with epilepsy (Goggin and Callaghan, 1985). Routine monitoring of serum clobazam levels is of limited value as there is large intersubject variability.

In animal models, clobazam has been shown to be effective against various seizure models in guinea-pigs, mice and baboons, including pentylenetetrazol, electroshock and reflex epilepsy (Barzaghi et al., 1973; Ballabio et al., 1981).

Steru et al. (1986) compared the anxiolytic, anticonvulsant, sedative and myorelaxant effects of several benzodiazepines in mice. Clobazam, when compared with the standard 1,4-benzodiazepines, had a superior anticonvulsant specificity with minimal sedative properties. It was eight to ten times less potent than diazepam in producing sedation, ataxia and muscle relaxation.

## ANTICONVULSANT EFFECTS OF CLOBAZAM

The first clinical report was that of Gastaut in 1978. He noted powerful anticonvulsant effects of clobazam given as adjunctive therapy for refractory seizures and commented that the improvement was of 'a percentage that has so far never been obtained with any other antiepileptic agent' (Gastaut, 1978). In a later report clobazam was reported to be rapidly effective and useful against all varieties of epileptic seizures in over half of the subjects treated (Gastaut and Low, 1979). Only mild adverse effects were noted, but tolerance to the anticonvulsant properties was recorded in a third of cases.

There are many open studies of clobazam in a variety of seizure types, which have been well reviewed by Robertson (1986). These include 22 published open trials, in a total of 880 patients aged six months to 69 years. The dose of clobazam used ranged from 10 mg to 130 mg. In the majority, clobazam was given as adjuvant medication, although in two studies clobazam was used as monotherapy in children (Dulac et al., 1983; Plouin and Jalin, 1985). Recently two extensive open studies have been reported, one from Australia and one from Canada.

A summary of the data from open studies is as follows: the improvement in seizure frequency ranged from 38% to 95% with a mean of 65%. The number of patients seizure-free, where it was reported, was 30%.

In the Australian study, Buchanan (1993) examined 56 patients aged 6 months to 59 years with a variety of seizure types. All were receiving other anticonvulsants, and follow-up was from one month to eight years. They reported 14 patients who had their seizures completely eradicated, with a greater than 50% reduction of seizures in 27 patients (48.2%).

In the Canadian study (Guberman et al., 1990), 80 adult patients were followed prospectively for an average of 14 months. This was combined with a retrospective survey of 424 adult patients followed up to six years who had been treated with clobazam. In the prospective study, 35.5% of patients remained on the drug at follow-up with a greater than 75% seizure reduction, and in the retrospective study it was shown that approximately 50% of adults obtained seizure improvement of more than 50%. Over a mean follow-up period of 18 months nearly 20% of patients were seizure-free, or almost seizure-free. Survival analysis in the retrospective study showed that nearly 45% of patients were still receiving clobazam after four years.

There have been five double-blind investigations and one single-blind study of clobazam in epilepsy. Critchley et al. (1981) reported on 27 patients with resistant seizures who were receiving maximum doses of one or more standard anticonvulsant drugs. They were given 20 mg of clobazam at night in a double-blind, cross-over trial against placebo. Eighteen of the 27 patients had fewer seizures on clobazam than placebo, six had more seizures, and three showed no change. Six patients became seizure-free.

Feely et al., (1982) gave 20–30 mg of clobazam daily as adjunctive therapy to 18 patients with catamenial epilepsy, comparing it with placebo over predetermined 10-day periods in a double-blind, cross-over design. Their results were evaluated by either complete cessation of catamenial seizures in patients usually having fewer than four seizures in a 10-day period, or a greater than 50% reduction of seizures in patients having more than four seizures in this time period. In 14 of the patients clobazam was superior to placebo, and in four no preference was established.

Allen *et al.* (1983) reported on 26 patients having four or more uncontrolled seizures a month who had tried standard anticonvulsant drugs. A dose of 30 mg of clobazam or placebo was prescribed at night as adjunctive therapy in a double-blind, cross-over trial for nine weeks. An eight-week washout period was allowed between treatments. The results showed a significant decrease in seizure frequency during the clobazam period, especially for partial seizures, and three patients became seizure-free.

Dellaportas *et al.* (1984) reported a double-blind comparison of two doses of clobazam (10 mg or 20 mg) against placebo on 31 patients whose seizures were still uncontrolled following adequate standard anticonvulsant drug therapy. The patients were followed six months prior to entering and were randomized into three groups according to their treatment regimen, being followed up for a further six months. The two clobazam groups showed a significant improvement compared with the placebo group. The improvement seemed to apply to both generalized and partial seizures, although the numbers having generalized seizures were small.

Aucamp (1985) studied 12 institutionalized epileptic patients with uncontrolled seizures in a cross-over design trial over a nine-week period with a five-week washout, comparing clobazam (0.5 mg/kg per day) against placebo. Nine patients became seizure-free, and a significant improvement was noted for severity of seizures, duration of seizures and frequency of seizures on the active drug.

The single-blind study was conducted by Del Pesce *et al.* (1979), in which clobazam was given over a 10-week period to a group of 28 patients, comparing it with placebo as adjunctive therapy. The anticonvulsant effect of clobazam was significantly better than that of placebo.

The conclusions from the double-blind trials are that clobazam clearly exerts a powerful anticonvulsant effect, often rendering patients seizure-free, which in a number of patients is sustained for the duration of the trial.

Several investigators have examined patients on clobazam for long periods of time. Martin (1985) followed a cohort of patients with resistant epilepsy for up to four years. Thirty-four per cent of 48 patients remained seizure-free for one to four years. Patients who remained seizure-free for such times received 10–50 mg of clobazam daily, the majority having 10–30 mg. Wolf (1985) added 10–20 mg to the therapy of 34 patients with intractable seizures, increasing by 10 mg doses until adverse effects appeared or seizures were controlled. On follow-up seven remained on the drug, five on account of continuing seizure control, and two because of psychotropic effects. Goggin and Callaghan (1985) gave 34 patients clobazam added to their existing therapy; 39% of cases maintained excellent or good control of seizures up to 12 months.

Heller *et al.* (1988) analysed the factors that related to a good response with clobazam in refractory epilepsy. Twenty-five out of 41 patients showed a dramatic response, nine cases maintaining this for a year. A known aetiology for the epilepsy, the occurrence of complex partial seizures alone, and absence of mental retardation were all related to a good outcome.

In the Australian study (Buchanan, 1993), a reduction of seizures (mean 65%, range 20–90%) lasted in some patients up to eight years (mean 3.4 years) and 14 patients (25%) were seizure-free. Patients with partial seizures responded better, and those with mental handicap fared worst. In the Canadian studies, 21% had a sustained improvement. A small group of patients were on monotherapy (seven) and they did less well than those on polytherapy. It was suggested that this may be due to increased levels of *N*-desmethylclobazam, which tends to be higher in patients on polytherapy with anticonvulsants that induce hepatic enzymes.

Data from the long-term studies, therefore, suggest that if patients continue on the drug beyond a three-month period, many of them are likely to be on the medication several years later. In the region of 10% of patients maintained on clobazam become seizure-free, a remarkable figure considering that the trials are carried out using patients in whom seizure control with standard anticonvulsants has failed. In the Canadian studies, 40–50% of patients were still taking clobazam after four years.

## SIDE-EFFECTS

Clobazam is relatively well tolerated and provokes fewer adverse effects than the 1,4-benzodiazepines. The most common side-effects are sedation, irritability, disinhibition, depression, ataxia and muscle weakness. Others include weight gain, psychosis, tremor, increased bronchial secretions, dizziness and insomnia. In some patients an increase in seizures is reported, particularly partial seizures.

Adverse effects are reported in 8–50% of patients, depending on the series, but only a total of 4% of patients had to be withdrawn from controlled or open studies because of side-effects (Robertson, 1986).

## PSYCHOTROPIC EFFECTS

In contrast, a number of studies have reported an improvement of patients' well-being, noting psychomotor arousal, improved attention and alertness, decreased anxiety, and a reduction of behaviour disorders such as impulsivity and aggression (Hindmarch, 1985). In some patients, this was due to the withdrawal of other benzodiazepines or other anticonvulsant drugs with a more toxic profile. However, there is evidence (Gastaut, 1981; Martin, 1981) suggesting that clobazam is better than the 1,4-benzodiazepines in relation to cognitive problems, and may indeed have some psychotropic effects (Hindmarch, 1985).

Scott and Moffett (1986) gave clobazam to 30 patients with epilepsy and noted fit frequency to be markedly reduced. They also administered psychological tests including the Middlesex Hospital questionnaire, the Stroop test, a stress anxiety questionnaire and visual analogue scales for mood. Performance on the Stroop test improved, as did the rating of psychopathology on the Middlesex Hospital questionnaire. On 15 visual analogue scales, all but one indicated a significant benefit for clobazam.

Cull and Trimble (1985) compared the effects of clobazam (10 mg three times a day) for two weeks and placebo in 10 healthy volunteers, contrasting this with the effects of clonazepam (0.5 mg three times a day) for two weeks versus placebo using a double-blind, cross-over design. Minimal impairment was found with clobazam in contrast to clonazepam, which affected a broad range of cognitive functions.

## PHARMACOKINETIC INTERACTIONS

Following the administration of clobazam, no significant changes are noted in carbamazepine, phenobarbitone or phenytoin serum levels (Allen et al., 1983; Wolf, 1985). However, in individual studies, interactions have been noted, such as an increase in valproate levels in healthy volunteers (Cocks et al., 1985), and increases in carbamazepine levels, which in some cases required dose reduction (Franceschi et al., 1983).

In contrast, carbamazepine and phenytoin raise levels of N-desmethylclobazam and lead to lower serum clobazam levels (Cano et al., 1981). No relationship has been found between serum clobazam or desmethylclobazam levels and clinical response, although it has been suggested that signs of toxicity are likely to develop if the clobazam level is greater than 0.6 µg/ml and the N-desmethylclobazam level is greater than 9 µg/ml.

## THE CLINICAL USE OF CLOBAZAM

Clobazam has been used clinically to treat a wide spectrum of seizure disorders in both children and adults. It has also been used satisfactorily as short-term treatment in catamenial epilepsy and other paroxysmal exacerbations of seizures. Because of its low toxicity profile and possible psychotropic effects, it may be useful in patients with epilepsy accompanied by behavioural disorders.

Advantages of the use of clobazam as an anticonvulsant include its high therapeutic index, and relatively broad spectrum of action across a wide range of seizure types. Because it has a long half-life it can be given in single daily doses. Benzodiazepines are known to have low levels of toxicity, their safety profile having been established over many years. Clobazam is safe in both children and adults, in children probably being of most value in the Lennox–Gastaut syndrome, and in those with uncontrolled atypical absence seizures, akinetic seizure and myoclonic seizures. In adults it is patients with complex partial seizures and secondary generalized seizures that respond best, probably where there is an identifiable cause for the epilepsy.

In clinical practice, clobazam has been advocated as adjunctive therapy. Indeed, in today's terms, this may represent one form of rational polypharmacy, where a drug with a clearly different structure from the conventional anticonvulsants is added to achieve a combined pharmacodynamic effect.

The main reported problem is that of tolerance, but the figures on this vary considerably between studies. Thus, in the review of Robertson (1986) the incidence ranges from 0% to 86%, with a mean of 36%. The Canadian experience was far lower (9.2%), and in the study of Buchanan (1993) 19.6% of patients developed tolerance. There are a number of reasons for these varying results, including different definitions of tolerance, failure to monitor compliance, and dosing schedules. The mechanism of the tolerance remains unknown.

From a practical point of view, tolerance usually develops within the first three months of treatment, and, although it may occur at any time beyond that, it appears to be the case that a high percentage of patients started on clobazam remain on the drug after several years. Once tolerance develops, clinical experience suggests that the clobazam needs to be withdrawn.

It is recommended that clobazam be given once or twice daily, starting at a 10 mg dose, increasing to 20 mg or beyond at weekly intervals. It can be given as a single night-time dose. In some countries a 5 mg dose is available, and is useful for children. The rate of increase depends on the other anticonvulsants patients are receiving, and the development of any possible side-effects.

Clobazam is recommended as an add-on agent to additional drugs, although there is little experience of combinations of clobazam with the new anticonvulsants that are described in other chapters of this book. It has been used satisfactorily as short-term treatment for catamenial epilepsy, or for other patients who have predictable paroxysmal exacerbations of seizures, with clusters. It may also be used to abort a bout of non-convulsive status, or to prevent the train of seizures in a known pattern of clusters, the patient being instructed to take the drug immediately after the first or second seizure of the cluster. Because of its low toxicity profile and possible psychotropic effects, it is also of value in patients who have accompanying behaviour disorders. There are no reports of patients with epilepsy developing dependency.

Clinical experience suggests that patients usually respond to low doses, but a few need higher doses. In some patients, complex partial seizures with behaviour automatisms may have their behavioural expression altered, by the use of higher doses, to become simple partial seizures, which are much less troublesome to patients. In other words, although no change in seizure frequency may be reported, seizure severity is improved. Doses as high as 80–100 mg are sometimes used, but in the majority of patients 10–20 mg is sufficient.

Adverse reactions, if they occur, usually begin within a few days of starting the drugs, although idiosyncratic adverse effects with some of the other anticonvulsant drugs, such as carbamazepine, may take several weeks to emerge.

It is important to warn patients prior to treatment that the drug may have an excellent initial effect, which may then wear off. It should be clearly stated that they need to give the drug at least three months before the true effect can be evaluated, and that even then in some patients the effect may wane. Avoidance of disappointment is important here.

As with all benzodiazepines, withdrawal seizures may be a problem if the drug is too rapidly discontinued. However, the long half-life, particularly of the desmethylclobazam metabolite, may exert a helpful protective effect, but generally slow withdrawal is recommended.

## CONCLUSION

In the oral management of seizures, clobazam represents an important advance on the 1,4-benzodiazepines, showing less in the way of toxicity, some psychotropic effects and a more sustained effect on seizures of various types. Generally the drug is well tolerated, and adverse effects are minimal.

When clobazam is used as adjunctive therapy in resistant patients, some 10–20% of patients will achieve a lasting benefit, often remaining seizure-free. In that these patients are resistant to conventional therapies, this represents a substantial treatment advance.

## REFERENCES

Allen JW, Oxley J, Robertson MM, Trimble MR, Richens A and Jawad SSM (1983) Clobazam as adjunctive treatment in refractory epilepsy. *Br. Med. J.*, **286**, 1246–1247.

Aucamp AK (1985) Clobazam as adjunctive therapy in uncontrolled epileptic patients. *Curr. Ther. Res.*, **37**, 1098–1103.

Ballabio M, Caccia S, Garattini S *et al.* (1981) Antiepileptic activity and kinetics of clobazam and N-desmethylclobazam in the guinea pig. *Arch. Int. Pharmacodyn.*, **253**, 192–199.

Barzaghi F, Fournex R and Mantegazza P (1973) Pharmacological and toxicological properties of clobazam (1-phenyl-5-methyl-8-chloro-1,2,4,5-tetrahydro-2,4-

diketo-3H-1,5-benzodiazepine), a new psychotherapeutic agent. *Arzneim. Forsch.,* **23**, 683–686.

Buchanan N (1993) Clobazam in the treatment of epilepsy: prospective follow up to eight years. *J. Roy. Soc. Med.,* **86**, 378–380.

Cano JP, Brun H, Iliadis A, Davet C, Roger J and Gastaut H (1981) Influence of antiepileptic drugs on plasma levels of clobazam and desmethylclobazam: application of research on relations between doses, plasma levels and clinical efficacy. In: *Clobazam* (eds I Hindmarch and PD Stonier), International Congress and Symposium Series No. 43, pp. 169–174. Royal Society of Medicine, London.

Cocks A, Critchley EMR, Hayward HW and Thomas D (1985) The effect of clobazam on the blood levels of sodium valproate. In: *Clobazam: Human Psychopharmacology and Clinical Applications* (eds I Hindmarch, PD Stonier and MR Trimble), International Congress and Symposium Series No. 74, pp. 155–157. Royal Society of Medicine, London.

Critchley EMR, Vakil SD, Hayward HW, Owen MVH, Cocks A and Freemantle NP (1981) Double-blind clinical trial of clobazam in refractory epilepsy. In: *Clobazam* (eds I Hindmarch and PD Stonier), International Congress and Symposium Series No. 43, pp. 159–163. Royal Society of Medicine, London.

Cull CA and Trimble MR (1985) Anticonvulsant benzodiazepines and performance. In: *Clobazam: Human Psychopharmacology and Clinical Applications* (eds I Hindmarch, PD Stonier and MR Trimble), International Congress and Symposium Series No. 74, pp. 121–128. Royal Society of Medicine, London.

Del Pesce M, Fua P, Fiuliani G, Provinciali L, Pigini P and Gamba G (1979) Clobazam as an antiepileptic drug. A controlled clinical trial of its efficacy, plasma levels and side effects in partial and secondary generalised epilepsy. In: *11th Epilepsy International Symposium,* Florence, Abstracts p. 423.

Dellaportas CI, Wilson A and Clifford Rose F (1984) Clobazam as adjunctive treatment in chronic epilepsy. In: *Advances in Epileptology: The XVth Epilepsy International Symposium* (eds RJ Porter, RH Mattson, AA Ward Jr and N Dam), pp. 363–367. Raven Press, New York.

Dulac O, Figueroa D, Rey E and Arthuis M (1983) Monotherapie par le clobazam dans les epilepsies de l'enfant. *Presse Med.* **12**, 1067–1069.

Feely M, Calvert R and Gibson J (1982) Clobazam in catamenial epilepsy: a model for evaluating anticonvulsants. *Lancet,* **ii**, 71–73.

Franceschi M, Ferini-Strambi L, Mastrangelo M and Smirne S (1983) Clobazam in drug-resistant and alcoholic withdrawal seizures. *Clin. Trials J.,* **20**, 119–125.

Gastaut H (1978) Proprietés antiepileptiques exceptionneles et meconnues d'un anxiolytique du commerce, le clobazam. *Concours Med.,* **100**, 3697–3701.

Gastaut H and Low MD (1979) Antiepileptic properties of clobazam, a 1,5 benzodiazepine, in man. *Epilepsia,* **20**, 437–446.

Gastaut H (1981) The effect of benzodiazepines on chronic epilepsy in man (with particular reference to clobazam). In: *Clobazam* (eds I Hindmarch and PD Stonier), International Congress and Symposium Series No. 43, pp. 141–150. Royal Society of Medicine, London.

Goggin T and Callaghan N (1985) Blood levels of clobazam and its metabolites and therapeutic effect. In: *Clobazam* (eds I Hindmarch, PD Stonier and MR Trimble), International Congress and Symposium Series No. 74, pp. 149–153. Royal Society of Medicine, London.

Guberman A, Couture M, Blaschuk K and Sherwin A (1990) Add-on trial of clobazam in intractable adult epilepsy with plasma level concentrations. *Can. J. Neurol. Sci.,* **17**, 311–316.

Heller AJ, Ring HA and Reynolds EG (1988) Factors relating to dramatic response to clobazam therapy in refractory epilepsy. *Epilepsy Res.*, **2**, 276–278.

Hindmarch I (1985) The psychopharmacology of clobazam. In: *Clobazam: Human Psychopharmacology and Clinical Applications* (eds I Hindmarch, PD Stonier and MR Trimble), International Congress and Symposium Series No. 74, pp. 3–10. Royal Society of Medicine, London.

Martin AA (1981) The antiepileptic effects of clobazam: a long-term study in resistant epilepsy. In: *Clobazam* (eds I Hindmarch and PD Stonier), International Congress and Symposium Series No. 43, pp. 151–157. Royal Society of Medicine, London.

Martin AA (1985) Clobazam in resistant epilepsy — a long-term study. In: *Clobazam: Human Psychopharmacology and Clinical Applications* (eds I Hindmarch, PD Stonier and MR Trimble), International Congress and Symposium Series No. 74, pp. 137–138. Royal Society of Medicine, London.

Plouin P and Jalin C (1985) EEG changes in epileptic children treated with clobazam as monotherapy. In: *Clobazam: Human Psychopharmacology and Clinical Applications* (eds I Hindmarch, PD Stonier and MR Trimble), International Congress and Symposium Series No. 74, pp. 191–197. Royal Society of Medicine, London.

Robertson MM (1986) Current status of the 1,4- and 1,5-benzodiazepines in the treatment of epilepsy. *Epilepsia*, **27**, (Suppl. 1) S27–S41.

Rupp W, Badian M, Christ O *et al.* (1979) Pharmacokinetics of single and multiple doses of clobazam in humans. *Br. J. Clin. Pharmacol.*, **7**, 51–57.

Scott DF and Moffett A (1986) On the anticonvulsant and psychotropic properties of clobazam — a preliminary study. *Epilepsia*, **27** (suppl. 1), 42–44.

Steru L, Chermat R, Millet B, Mico JA and Simon P (1986) Comparative study in mice of 10 1,4 benzodiazepines and of clobazam: anticonvulsant, anxiolytic, sedative, and myorelaxant effects. *Epilepsia*, **27** (suppl. 1), 14–17.

Wolf P (1985) Clobazam in drug-resistant patients with complex focal seizures — report of an open study. In: *Clobazam: Human Psychopharmacology and Clinical Applications* (eds Hindmarch I, PD Stonier and MR Trimble), International Congress and Symposium Series No. 74, pp. 167–171. Royal Society of Medicine, London.

# 4

# Felbamate

W. Edwin Dodson
*Washington University School of Medicine, St Louis, Missouri, USA*

## INTRODUCTION

Felbamate is a new anticonvulsant drug that was approved by the United States Food and Drug Administration in August 1993, approximately 15 years after the approval of valproate. Its authorization was based on several novel approaches to demonstrating its anticonvulsant efficacy. Felbamate is effective against partial and partial secondarily generalized seizures and in the Lennox–Gastaut syndrome.

### Chemistry and Metabolism

Felbamate (2-phenyl-1,3-propanediol dicarbamate) is chemically related to meprobamate, but unlike meprobamate felbamate lacks anxiolytic and muscle relaxant properties. The anticonvulsant properties of felbamate were discovered in the empirical screening programme sponsored by the Antiepileptic Drug Development Program at the National Institutes of Health (Swinyard *et al.*, 1986, 1987; White *et al.*, 1992). It can be measured in small serum samples by high-performance liquid chromatography simultaneously with other anticonvulsants (Remmel *et al.*, 1990; Clark *et al.*, 1992).

Approximately half of administered doses is excreted unchanged in urine and the reminder is metabolized to the *p*-hydroxy (2-(4-hydroxyphenyl)-1,3-propanediol dicarbamate) and 2-hydroxy (2-hydroxy-2-phenyl-1,3-propanediol dicarbamate) metabolites in mice, rats, rabbits and dogs (Adusumalli *et al.*, 1991; Yang *et al.*, 1991; Bialer, 1993).

*New Anticonvulsants: Advances in the Treatment of Epilepsy.* Edited by M. R. Trimble
© 1994 John Wiley & Sons Ltd

## Spectrum of activity in animal models

Animal studies have shown felbamate to have a broad spectrum of anticonvulsant activity similar to phenobarbitone and valproate. The mechanism of action of felbamate is unknown, but it is active in several experimental models of epilepsy (Macdonald and Kelly, 1993). In rodents felbamate is effective against seizures induced by maximal electroshock and by chemoconvulsants (Swinyard *et al.*, 1986, 1987; Gordon *et al.*, 1991). There has been no evidence of tolerance to its actions against experimentally induced seizures in animals (Swinyard *et al.*, 1987).

Compared with standard anticonvulsant drugs, felbamate had a higher protective index (the median toxic dose divided by the median effective dose) against seizures induced by maximal electroshock in rats and mice (Swinyard *et al.*, 1986, 1987). Furthermore, in rodents, felbamate potentiates the protective effects of phenytoin, carbamazepine, valproate and phenobarbitone against seizures induced by maximal electroshock. Interestingly, this potentiation occurs without additive rotorod toxicity, resulting in an increased protective index for these combinations in rodents (Gordon *et al.*, 1993).

Like phenytoin, felbamate prevents sustained repetitive firing in cultured mouse spinal neurons with a median inhibitory concentration of 67 mg/l (White *et al.*, 1992). Although this suggests similar mechanisms of action, clearly the two compounds act differently, because felbamate is effective against pentylenetetrazol-induced seizures whereas phenytoin is not.

Felbamate prevents experimental seizures induced by various chemicals including pentylenetetrazol (Metrazol) (Swinyard *et al.*, 1987; Gordon *et al.*, 1991). Felbamate is also active against seizures caused by isoniazid but not against seizures caused by bicuculline and strychnine (Swinyard *et al.*, 1986; Gordon *et al.*, 1991). Felbamate enhanced the action of diazepam against maximal electroshock, pentylenetetrazol and isoniazid but not bicuculline. Despite this interaction, felbamate may not appear to act at the gamma-aminobutyric acid (GABA) receptor complex because it does not alter the binding of various ligands to the receptor complex (Ticku *et al.*, 1991). It is also effective against pilocarpine-induced seizures in rodents after lithium pretreatment, more so than in lithium-free animals (Sofia *et al.*, 1993).

Like phenytoin, carbamazepine, zonisamide, phenobarbitone and valproate, felbamate also protects against lethal seizures induced by 4-aminopyridine, a potassium channel blocker. Anticonvulsant drugs such as diazepam, vigabatrin and tiagabine, which act by potentiating endogenously released GABA are ineffective in this model, as are ethosuximide, nimodipine and certain *N*-methyl-D-aspartate (NMDA) antagonists such as MK-801 (Yamaguchi and Rogawski, 1992).

Felbamate is also effective in kainic acid-induced status in 30-day-old rats. When tested 80 days later, felbamate-treated rats did better on the water maze test of learning and had longer latencies against flurothyl-induced seizures than rats which had previously been treated with placebo and had experienced longer seizures (Chronopoulos *et al.*, 1993). This and other experiments have indicated so-called neuroprotective effects.

Several studies have suggested that felbamate has neuroprotective actions against kainic acid-induced seizures and experimental models of hypoxia–ischaemia (Wasterlain *et al.*, 1992; McCabe *et al.*, 1993). In mice, felbamate prevents clonus induced by intraventricular injected NMDA and tonic forelimb extension induced by quisqualic acid administered similarly. It also prevents stage 5 seizures in electrically kindled mice (White *et al.*, 1992). In another study, felbamate in concentrations at or above 45 mg/l protected CA-1 neurons in hippocampal slices against hypoxia (Wallis *et al.*, 1992).

Combining the results of various efficacy models with the rotorod neurotoxicity test demonstrated that felbamate has a very high protective index of 28 to 146 (White *et al.*, 1992).

Thus, felbamate appears to have a unique mechanism of action and a broad spectrum of activity in various animal seizure models. Compared with other anticonvulsant drugs in experimental animals it has one of the highest protective indices, which forecasts good acute tolerability. Even though its precise mechanism of action has not yet been elucidated, felbamate's activity against both maximal electroshock and pentylenetetrazol in screening models correlates with a broad spectrum of anticonvulsant potential in humans.

## CLINICAL INDICATIONS

Indications for felbamate include partial and secondarily generalized seizures and partial, astatic and generalized tonic–clonic seizures in children. Currently, experience with felbamate is most extensive in patients with severe epilepsy who have partial and partial secondarily generalized seizures, as well as children with Lennox–Gastaut syndrome. Among these types of difficult-to-treat patients, 50% of them have had a 50% or greater reduction in seizure frequency.

Novel study designs to demonstrate felbamate's efficacy were used in its development. Because these studies had end-points that differed from the customary end-point of seizure frequency, there is actually little information available about the percentage of subjects whose epilepsy responds in comparison with more traditional studies of other drugs.

A little background information is helpful in understanding the strategy for the development of felbamate. In May 1988, a meeting was held at the National Institutes of Health (NIH) to consider the design of clinical studies for investigating new anticonvulsant drugs. Sponsored by the Epilepsy Branch at NIH, the meeting convened academic investigators and representatives of government-sponsored anticonvulsant drug development programmes; the pharmaceutical industry and the Food and Drug Administration (G.W. Pledger, personal communication, 1988). Regulatory representatives affirmed that in order for studies to be accepted as evidence for approval in the USA, they need to show a difference either in the form of a dose–response relationship, or between the investigational drug and another agent. Further discussions emphasized the need to use patients less therapy-resistant, to begin monotherapy trials, to consider brief placebo trials with rescue provisions, to use patients with high seizure frequencies such as patients undergoing presurgical monitoring, and to conduct investigations of new drugs in children.

Several of these recommendations were incorporated into the clinical studies that demonstrated the anticonvulsant efficacy of felbamate, notably the use of presurgical patients, trials of monotherapy with rescue provisions comparing felbamate with low-dose active control (valproate) and the evaluation of felbamate in children with the Lennox–Gastaut syndrome.

## FELBAMATE IN PARTIAL AND GENERALIZED TONIC–CLONIC SEIZURES

One of the first published studies of felbamate was a double-blind, randomized, placebo-controlled trial in subjects with partial seizures (Leppik *et al.*, 1991). Inclusion criteria included four or more partial seizures per month despite concomitant therapeutic blood levels of phenytoin plus carbamazepine. Fifty-six adult patients were enrolled in this add-on study. Felbamate was statistically superior to placebo in several aspects including seizure reduction, percentage seizure reduction, and truncated percentage seizure reduction. The average dose of felbamate was 2300 mg per day, somewhat lower than in subsequent studies.

In a similar add-on study where the maximal dose was 3000 mg per day, the difference between felbamate and placebo was not statistically significant (Theodore *et al.*, 1991). However, felbamate also lowered carbamazepine levels; when this was taken into account the results suggested the efficacy of felbamate. Both of these early add-on studies used lower doses than subsequent monotherapy trials where the dose was 3600 mg per day.

In two studies among outpatients, felbamate given alone was shown to be effective in comparison with low-dose valproate (Sachdeo *et al.*, 1992; Faught *et al.*, 1993). The first published study (Sachdeo *et al.*, 1992) enrolled 44 subjects with partial seizures on monotherapy who had eight or more seizures during a 56-day baseline period. At randomization, subjects were switched to either felbamate 3600 mg per day or valproate 15 mg/kg per day. The endpoint was either completion of the 112-day study period or achievement of 'escape criteria'. Escape criteria included a doubling of monthly seizure frequency, doubling of highest two-day seizure frequency, a single generalized tonic–clonic seizure if none had occurred during baseline, or significant prolongation of generalized tonic–clonic seizures. A significant advantage was seen for felbamate, with only three patients escaping versus 19 escaping on valproate.

In a similar but larger multicentre study, felbamate was confirmed to have efficacy against partial seizures (Faught et al., 1993). This investigation involved 111 subjects and had slightly different escape criteria, but the results were similar to the first. On felbamate significantly fewer subjects (18) achieved the criteria for escape as compared with subjects on valproate, of whom 37 escaped.

The anticonvulsant effect of felbamate also was demonstrated in patients who had their anticonvulsant drugs withdrawn as part of presurgical evaluations. After the patients were withdrawn from previous anticonvulsant drugs for the purpose of documenting their seizures, they underwent a randomized, placebo-controlled trial before resuming their pre-evaluation medication regimens. As expected, their seizure frequencies increased after anticonvulsant drugs were discontinued. The study lasted until the subjects had a fourth seizure or for a maximum of 28 days.

The presurgical trial enrolled 64 patients with partial seizures and partial secondarily generalized seizures (Bourgeois et al., 1993). After completing the videoelectroencephalographic monitoring, subjects were randomized to either felbamate 3600 mg per day or placebo. Doses of felbamate were titrated upward quickly over three days. The major outcome variable was the time to the fourth seizure. On placebo, 84% of subjects had a fourth seizure before the end of the 28-day study. On felbamate 46% had four seizures during the study period. Thus, only 16% of placebo patients completed the 28-day trial with four or fewer seizures, whereas 54% of subjects on felbamate successfully completed the 28-day period. After the study, all of the subjects resumed their previous medications.

## FELBAMATE IN LENNOX–GASTAUT SYNDROME

Felbamate is the first drug to be shown effective in randomized, controlled trials in the Lennox–Gastaut syndrome, one of the most severe forms of childhood epilepsy (Felbamate Study Group in Lennox–Gastaut Syndrome, 1993). In children with Lennox–Gastaut syndrome who had very high seizure frequencies, felbamate was tested against placebo in an add-on, randomized, double-blind trial in 73 subjects. At randomization, carbamazepine, phenytoin and valproate doses were reduced by 25% because of the previously discovered interactions of felbamate with these drugs.

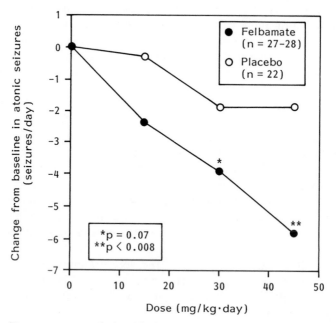

**Figure 1.**   Dose–response relationship between felbamate dose and reduction in frequency of astatic (atonic) seizure. Figure provided by Wallace Laboratories

Felbamate significantly reduced the frequencies of astatic seizures (drop attacks), generalized tonic–clonic seizures plus total seizure counts, but not atypical absence seizures. In addition, felbamate-treated subjects improved significantly more on a parent-rated single item of global evaluation. Significantly, felbamate-treated children had fewer injuries, substantiating the benefit of reducing astatic seizures. Overall, approximately 50% of these subjects experienced a 50% or greater reduction in total seizure frequency. Dose–response and concentration–response relationships were apparent against astatic seizures (Figure 1).

Following the randomized trial, all subjects were switched to felbamate as part of an open-label, follow-on investigation (Dodson, 1993). In the first month of open-label felbamate treatment, 62% of the subjects who previously took placebo had a reduction in total seizure frequency of greater than 50%. This response rate was similar to that in subjects who took felbamate during the double-blind study. Furthermore, the improvement that occurred in the double-blind study was sustained in the subsequent follow-on study for 12 months. Overall, approximately half of the patients had a 50% reduction in total seizure count by the 12-month follow-up point. Astatic seizures responded best, with two-thirds of patients having a reduction of more than 50% after 12 months' treatment (Figure 2). Although most subjects with

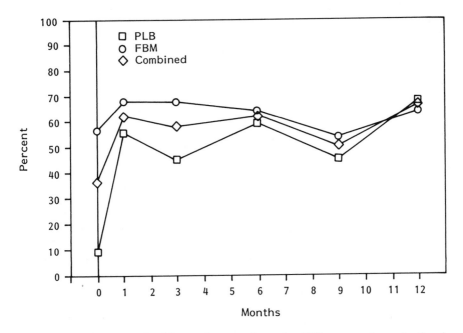

**Figure 2.** Percentage of subjects who experienced a 50% or greater reduction in astatic seizures in the randomized, controlled trial and the subsequent 12 months of open-label follow-on investigation. FBM, felbamate; PLB, placebo. Reproduced from Dodson (1993) with permission

Lennox–Gastaut syndrome did not become seizure-free, the frequency of their most severe seizure types decreased and their overall functioning improved due to enhanced alertness and responsiveness to their caretakers.

## PHARMACOKINETICS

Felbamate has predictable, linear elimination kinetics (Graves *et al.*, 1989a,b; Adusumalli *et al.*, 1991; Albani *et al.*, 1991) (Table 1). Distributed throughout the body, felbamate enters the brain rapidly where its initial localization is largely a function of regional cerebral blood flow (Cornford *et al.*, 1992). It is well absorbed after oral administration and peak concentrations occur in approximately four hours. Felbamate has a half-life in the range of 12–20 hours, with shorter values expected in children and those who take other drugs that induce hepatic drug metabolism. Thus, felbamate concentrations reach steady state in seven days or less unless there are concurrent drug interactions. The relationship between blood levels of felbamate and clinical response has not been characterized thus far, and a therapeutic range has not been defined.

**Table 1.**    Summary of felbamate pharmacokinetics

| | |
|---|---|
| Dose: | Adults 2400–3600 mg per day |
| | Children 30–60 mg/kg per day |
| Time to peak concentration ($t_{max}$): | 2–6 hours |
| Half-life ($t_{1/2}$): | 12–20 hours |
| Therapeutic range: | Undefined |
| Elimination: | Linear kinetics |
| | 50% metabolized in liver |
| | 50% excreted unchanged in urine |
| Drug interactions: | |
| *Affects* | Increases phenytoin, valproate and carbamazepine 10,11-epoxide |
| | Increases action of warfarin anticoagulants |
| | Decreases carbamazepine |
| *Affected by* | Decreased by phenytoin and carbamazepine |
| | Increased by valproate |

## DRUG INTERACTIONS

Felbamate is subject to both pharmacokinetic and pharmacodynamic interactions. The site of the pharmacokinetic interactions is the hepatic cytochrome P450 drug-metabolizing complex (Adusumalli *et al.*, 1991). Drug interactions involving felbamate are complex and operate both ways, as felbamate affects the clearance of other drugs while they simultaneously affect felbamate clearance (Table 1).

Felbamate increases the levels of phenytoin and valproate by inhibiting their hepatic metabolism. Stimulating hepatic metabolism, felbamate reduces carbamazepine levels slightly. However, it also seems to have an additive pharmacodynamic interaction with carbamazepine because side-effects have occurred in more than 90% of patients when carbamazepine was not reduced as felbamate was added (Fuerst *et al.*, 1988; Graves *et al.*, 1989a,b; Albani *et al.*, 1991; unpublished information on file, Wallace Laboratories). Usually, the felbamate-induced decrease in carbamazepine levels is modest but the range is fairly wide, with some patients experiencing a decline of more than 40% (Albani *et al.*, 1991; Wagner *et al.*, 1991). In one study the mean felbamate-induced reduction of carbamazepine levels was 1.3 µg/ml (5.5 µmol/l) (Graves *et al.*, 1989a). By inhibiting epoxide hydrolase, felbamate approximately doubles the ratio of carbamazepine 10,11-epoxide (CBZE) to carbamazepine. However, this interaction is probably of limited significance because CBZE levels are usually low, ranging from 10% of carbamazepine levels in patients on monotherapy to 50% among patients on polytherapy that includes phenytoin and valproate (Fuerst *et al.*, 1988; Wagner *et al.*, 1993).

Felbamate is not bound to serum constituents to a significant extent. Thus binding interactions involving felbamate are not expected and none has been observed (Albani *et al.*, 1991).

Thus far, felbamate has potentiated the action of coumadin in a single patient. This, in addition to the knowledge that felbamate inhibits hepatic cytochrome P450 drug-metabolizing enzymes, indicates that coagulation indices should be evaluated when felbamate is added to or deleted from drug regimens of patients who take warfarin anticoagulants.

Felbamate clearance is increased by interactions with carbamazepine, phenytoin and probably by phenobarbitone. Thus lower felbamate level to dose ratios are expected among patients who take felbamate with these anticonvulsants (Wagner *et al.*, 1991).

## ADVERSE EFFECTS

As predicted in animal studies of acute neurotoxicity, felbamate has a low incidence of side-effects and is well tolerated (Table 2). Idiosyncratic rashes are uncommon, occurring in less than 1% of exposed patients. Dose-related side-effects are also mild and infrequent, especially in monotherapy; however, as with other anticonvulsant drugs, side-effects are more frequent and can be troublesome in polytherapy. When this occurs, the side-effect usually ameliorates if the dose of co-medication is reduced.

The most frequent acute side-effects are gastrointestinal. These almost always abate with time or dosage reduction. Reduced appetite with weight loss infrequently is a problem in children but occasionally is welcomed by adult patients who are overweight. When weight loss occurs in children it is usually a transient concern as the weight decreases, stabilizes and then begins to increase over a period of several weeks to a few months. Rarely has it been necessary to stop felbamate therapy for this reason. The situation with insomnia is similar.

**Table 2.**   The most common adverse effects of felbamate reported during pre-approval studies. The percentages shown in parentheses were detected in patients on polytherapy. Side-effects are less frequent on monotherapy. (Based on data on file at Wallace Laboratories, 1992)

| Adults | Children |
| --- | --- |
| Nausea (11%) | Anorexia (6%) |
| Anorexia (7%) | Somnolence (6%) |
| Dizziness (6%) | Insomnia (6%) |
| Weight loss (4%) | Vomiting (3%) |
| Insomnia (4%) | Weight loss (2%) |

Insomnia is troublesome in children more often than in adults. Tricks for minimizing the impact of felbamate-induced insomnia include avoiding high doses one or two hours before bedtime, either by distributing more of the dose earlier in the day or by giving the dose as late as possible before retiring. Of course, intake of other compounds that interfere with falling asleep, such as caffeine and chocolate, should be restricted. Although some physicians recommend short-acting hypnotics to induce sleep onset in this situation, this is best avoided. As with other side-effects, most affected patients become tolerant and re-establish their previous sleep patterns within one or two weeks.

The risks of teratogenesis due to felbamate is unknown because experience in humans is limited. Pre-approval animal studies suggest that the risk in humans should be no greater than with traditional anticonvulsants.

## PRINCIPLES OF DOSING WITH FELBAMATE

Felbamate doses should be adjusted according to the patient's clinical response. This means that patients should start at low or average doses which should be increased stepwise until either seizures are controlled or intolerable side-effects occur. Felbamate levels have not been used to adjust felbamate dosing thus far and do not appear to be necessary based on clinical experience to date. In pre-approval efficacy studies, doses ranged up to 3600 mg per day in adults and to 45 mg/kg per day in children. Tolerability studies included doses of up to 60 mg/kg per day.

Initially the recommendation for a starting dose in adults was 1200 mg per day in two or three divided doses but based on more experience, lower starting doses of 600 or 900 mg per day are better tolerated. Unless frequent seizures make it necessary to increase the dose rapidly, increase the dose at intervals of two or more weeks as indicated by the patient's clinical response. Note that rapid upward titration of the dose in three days or less has been used in presurgical patients with high seizure frequencies, but a slower rate reduces the chance of acute side-effects, especially gastrointestinal upset. In children, weekly dosage increments of 15 mg/kg per day were tolerated well when felbamate was added to or substituted for other anticonvulsant drugs. Begin with 15 mg/kg per day and increase to 30, 45 or 60 mg/kg per day depending on the clinical situation and the child's response.

When felbamate is added to the regimens of patients who take other drugs, the best way to avoid side-effects is to reduce the doses of the other drugs when felbamate is started (Table 3). In order to maintain constant phenytoin and valproate levels when felbamate is added, it is necessary to reduce the phenytoin and valproate doses by 10–30%. Although there has been concern about precipitating severe or prolonged seizures by reducing these co-medications, this has not been observed thus far. In addition, it is usually wise

**Table 3.** A proposed schedule for substituting felbamate for carbamazepine, phenytoin or valproate. Visits occur every 7 to 21 days or as dictated by the severity of the patient's condition. At each visit the patient should be evaluated clinically and the schedule modified as indicated by the patient's situation. Replacing barbiturates and benzodiazepines with felbamate should be done more slowly and cautiously

| | |
|---|---|
| First visit | Start felbamate at 800 to 1200 mg per day (15 mg/kg per day for children) in divided doses. Reduce carbamazepine, phenytoin or valproate by 25–33% |
| Second visit | Increase felbamate to 1200 to 2400 mg per day (30 mg/kg per day in children). Reduce the drug targeted for replacement to one-third of the original dose |
| Third visit | Increase felbamate to 2400 to 3600 mg per day (45 mg/kg per day in children). Discontinue the drug targeted for replacement |
| Fourth visit | Revaluate the patient and adjust medications as indicated clinically |

to reduce the dose of carbamazepine by approximately 25% in order to avoid side-effects even though felbamate slightly reduces carbamazepine levels.

If side-effects occur while felbamate is being added to or substituted for other anticonvulsant drugs, clinical experience indicates that the better course of action is usually to accelerate the reduction of the co-medication rather than reduce the dose of felbamate. Although substitution of felbamate for carbamazepine, phenytoin and valproate can be accomplished in three weeks or less, starting with lower doses and making the transition more slowly reduces the chance of side-effects. While the experience with these three drugs is substantial, the experience with barbiturates and benzodiazepines is limited and should be regarded as preliminary. For this reason felbamate should be substituted for barbiturates and especially benzodiazepines cautiously and more slowly.

## CONCLUSION

Felbamate is a welcome addition to the treatment of epilepsy. In particular it is an important innovation for the treatment of refractory partial epilepsies and severe childhood epilepsy with astatic, partial and generalized tonic–clonic seizures. Clinically significant side-effects are uncommon and the drug is well tolerated by most patients. In fact, many patients who have taken it without significant reduction in seizure frequency have elected to continue it because of the relative lack of side-effects. Life-threatening or otherwise serious side-effects such as exfoliative rashes appear to be very rare indeed. No adverse effects on haematopoietic, hepatic or renal function have been noted.

The principal negative feature of felbamate is its extensive range of drug interactions. However, the impact of these can be minimized by prospective reductions in co-medications when felbamate is started. Much remains to be learned about this new drug before its place in the therapy of epilepsy is established (Ramsey, 1991; Vajda, 1992). For example, it is not yet known whether it will be as helpful in primary generalized epilepsies as it has been in partial epilepsies. Similarly, its role in the treatment of new onset seizures is not yet defined, but its favourable toxicity profile indicates that it may prove worthwhile here as well.

# REFERENCES

Adusumalli VE, Wong KK, Kucharczyk N and Sofia RD (1991) Felbamate in vitro metabolism by rat liver microsomes. *Drug. Metab. Dispos.*, **19**, 1135–1138.

Albani F, Theodore WH, Washington P *et al.* (1991) Effect of felbamate on plasma levels of carbamazepine and its metabolites. *Epilepsia*, **32**, 130–132.

Bialer M (1993) Comparative pharmacokinetics of the newer antiepileptic drugs. *Clin. Pharmacokinet.*, **24**, 441–452.

Bourgeois B, Leppik IE, Sackellares JC *et al.* (1993) Felbamate: a double-blind controlled trial in patients undergoing presurgical evaluation of partial seizures. *Neurology*, **43**, 693–696.

Chronopoulos A, Stafstrom C, Thurber S, Hyde P, Mikati M and Holmes GL (1993) Neuroprotective effect of felbamate after kainic acid-induced status epilepticus. *Epilepsia*, **34**, 359–366.

Clark LA, Wichmann JK, Kucharczyk N and Sofia RD (1992) Determination of the anticonvulsant felbamate in beagle dog plasma by high-performance liquid chromatography. *J. Chromatogr.*, **573**, 113–119.

Cornford EM, Young D, Paxton JW and Sofia RD (1992) Blood-brain barrier penetration of felbamate. *Epilepsia*, **33**, 944–954.

Dodson WE (1993) Felbamate in the treatment of Lennox–Gastaut syndrome: twelve months follow-up experience after a randomized controlled trial of felbamate versus placebo. *Epilepsia*.

Faught E, Sachdeo RC, Remler MP *et al.* (1993) Felbamate monotherapy for partial-onset seizures: an active-control trial. *Neurology*, **43**, 688–692.

Felbamate Study Group in Lennox–Gastaut Syndrome (1993) Efficacy of felbamate in childhood epileptic encephalopathy (Lennox–Gastaut syndrome). *N. Eng. J. Med.*, **328**, 29–33.

Fuerst RH, Graves NM, Leppik IE, Brundage RC, Holmes GB and Remmel RP (1988) Felbamate increases phenytoin but decreases carbamazepine concentration. *Epilepsia*, **29**, 488–491.

Gordon R, Gels M, Diamantis W and Sofia RD (1991) Interaction of felbamate and diazepam against maximal electroshock seizures and chemoconvulsants in mice. *Pharmacol. Biochem. Behav.*, **40**, 109–113.

Gordon R, Gels M, Wichmann J, Diamantis W and Sofia RD (1993) Interaction of felbamate with several other antiepileptic drugs against seizures induced by maximal electroshock in mice. *Epilepsia*, **34**, 367–371.

Graves NM, Holmes GB, Fuerst RH and Leppik IE (1989a) Effect of felbamate on phenytoin and carbamazepine serum concentrations. *Epilepsia,* **30**, 225–229.

Graves NM, Ludden TM, Holmes GB, Fuerst RH and Leppik IE (1989b) Pharmacokinetics of felbamate, a novel antiepileptic drug: application of mixed-effect modeling to clinical trials. *Pharmacotherapy,* **9**, 372–376.

Leppik IE, Dreifuss FE, Pledger GW *et al.* (1991) Felbamate for partial seizures: results of a controlled clinical trial. *Neurology,* **4**, 1785–1789.

Macdonald RL and Kelly KM (1993) Antiepileptic drug mechanisms of action. *Epilepsia,* **34** (suppl. 5), S1–8.

McCabe RT, Wasterlain CG, Kucharczyk N, Sofia RD and Vogel JR (1993) Evidence for anticonvulsant and neuroprotectant action of felbamate mediated by strychnine-insensitive glycine receptors. *J. Pharmacol. Exp. Ther.,* **264**, 1248–1252.

Ramsay RE (1991) Advances in the pharmacotherapy of epilepsy. *Epilepsia,* **34** (suppl. 5), S9–16.

Remmel RP, Miller SA and Graves NM (1990) Simultaneous assay of felbamate plus carbamazepine, phenytoin, and their metabolites by liquid chromatography with mobile phase optimization. *Ther. Drug Monit.,* **12**, 90–96.

Sachdeo R, Kramer LD, Rosenberg A and Sachdeo S (1992) Felbamate monotherapy: controlled trial in patients with partial onset seizures. *Ann. Neurol.,* **32**, 386–392.

Sofia RD, Gordon R, Gels M and Diamantis W (1993) Effects of felbamate and other anticonvulsant drugs in two models of status epilepticus in the rat. *Res. Commun. Chem. Pathol. Pharmacol.,* **79**, 335–341.

Swinyard EA, Sofia RD and Kupferberg HJ (1986) Comparative anticonvulsant activity and neurotoxicity of felbamate and four prototype antiepileptic drugs in mice and rats. *Epilepsia,* **27**, 27–34.

Swinyard EA, Woodhead JH, Franklin MR, Sofia RD and Kupferberg HJ (1987) The effect of chronic felbamate administration on anticonvulsant activity and hepatic drug-metabolizing enzymes in mice and rats. *Epilepsia,* **28**, 295–300.

Theodore WH, Raubertas RF, Porter RJ *et al.* (1991) Felbamate: a clinical trial for complex partial seizures. *Epilepsia,* **32**, 392–397.

Ticku MK, Kamatchi GL and Sofia RD (1991) Effect of anticonvulsant felbamate on GABAA receptor system. *Epilepsia,* **32**, 389–391.

Vajda FJ (1992) New anticonvulsants. *Curr. Opin. Neurol. Neurosurg.,* **5**, 519–525.

Wagner ML, Graves NM, Marienau K, Holmes GB, Remmel RP and Leppik IE (1991) Discontinuation of phenytoin and carbamazepine in patients receiving felbamate. *Epilepsia,* **32**, 398–406.

Wagner ML, Remmel RP, Graves NM and Leppik IE (1993) Effect of felbamate on carbamazepine and its major metabolites. *Clin. Pharmacol. Therap.,* **53**, 536–543.

Wallis RA, Panizzon KL, Fairchild MD and Wasterlain CG (1992) Protective effects of felbamate against hypoxia in the rat hippocampal slice. *Stroke,* **23**, 547–551.

Wasterlain CG, Adams LM, Hattori H and Schwartz PH (1992) Felbamate reduces hypoxic-ischemic brain damage in vivo. *Eur. J. Pharmacol.,* **212**, 275–278.

White HS, Wolf HH, Swinyard EA, Skeen GA and Sofia RD (1992) A neuropharmacological evaluation of felbamate as a novel anticonvulsant. *Epilepsia,* **33**, 564–572.

Yamaguchi S and Rogawski MA (1992) Effects of anticonvulsant drugs on 4-aminopyridine-induced seizures in mice. *Epilepsy Res.,* **11**, 9–16.

Yang JT, Adusumalli VE, Wong KK, Kucharczyk N and Sofia RD (1991) Felbamate metabolism in the rat, rabbit, and dog. *Drug. Metab.,* **19**, 1126–1134.

# 5

# Gabapentin

DAVID CHADWICK
*Walton Centre for Neurology and Neurosurgery, Liverpool, UK*

## INTRODUCTION

Gabapentin is a chemically novel compound related in structure to the neurotransmitter gamma-aminobutyric acid (GABA), which has been developed by Warner-Lambert. Gabapentin was synthesized as a GABA mimetic that could freely cross the blood–brain barrier. Despite its structural relationship to GABA and its anticonvulsant activity, gabapentin does not appear to act pharmacologically as a GABA mimetic.

## CHEMISTRY

Gabapentin, 1-(aminomethyl)cyclohexaneacetic acid, has a molecular weight of 171.34, is freely soluble in water (over 10% at pH 7.4), and does not exist in enantiomeric forms (Bartoszyk *et al.*, 1986). In the crystalline state it is stable at room temperature, but a low formation of the lactam occurs in aqueous solutions. Gabapentin may be assayed in plasma and urine by sensitive high-performance liquid chromatography with pre-column labelling for ultraviolet detection (Hengy and Kolle, 1985).

## TOXICOLOGY

Gabapentin is well tolerated, with no deaths in acute dosage animal studies at dose up to 8000 mg per day in rats and up to 5000 mg per day in mice. Studies of chronic administration show similar good tolerance with doses up to 1500 mg per day in rats, up to 2000 mg per day in dogs and up to 500 mg per day in

*New Anticonvulsants: Advances in the Treatment of Epilepsy.* Edited by M. R. Trimble
© 1994 John Wiley & Sons Ltd

monkeys. Minor increases in liver enzymes and increased organ weights seen at the highest doses all reversed promptly after cessation of therapy. Gabapentin is not mutagenic in bacterial and mammalian assays and is not teratogenic in three animal species (Bartoszyk et al., 1986).

Toxicology data from two-year bioassay studies conducted in rats and mice show an increase in acinar cell carcinomas of the pancreas in male Wistar rats only. The tumours were not seen in female rats or mice of either sex. In the study, designed to evaluate carcinogenicity, male and female rats were given gabapentin at 250 mg/kg, 1000 mg/kg or 2000 mg/kg daily for two years. Mean plasma concentrations at these doses were 24.2 µg/ml, 51.2 µg/ml and 84.6 µg/ml, respectively. For reference, plasma concentrations from current clinical studies commonly range from 2 µg/ml up to peak concentrations of 15 µg/ml.

The clinical relevance of these data is uncertain but probably does not represent a significant clinical risk.

## PHARMACOLOGICAL PROPERTIES

Gabapentin has been shown to prevent seizures in several animal models and in clinical studies. It has a mechanism of action that appears to be different from other anticonvulsant drugs.

Originally, gabapentin was synthesized as a structural analogue of the inhibitory neurotransmitter GABA, with the idea that it would mimic the actions of GABA in the brain. Indeed, gabapentin consists of the same amino acid backbone as GABA, except with a cyclohexyl ring incorporated. It was thought that with the added carbohydrate bulk, gabapentin would be able to penetrate the blood–brain barrier, which GABA fails to do.

Although gabapentin does penetrate the blood–brain barrier effectively (Vollmer et al., 1986) and has anticonvulsant properties in vivo (Bartoszyk et al., 1986), it does not interact with $GABA_A$ or $GABA_B$ receptors, nor is it converted metabolically into GABA or a GABA agonist. It is not an inhibitor of GABA uptake nor of degradation by GABA transaminase at relevant concentrations. However, at doses that prevent electroshock seizures in rats, it increases GABA accumulation induced by amino-oxyacetic acid in several regions of rat brain, but the molecular mechanisms of this effect is not known (Loscher et al., 1991). Therefore, gabapentin cannot be described as GABA mimetic, and despite activity in a variety of models, in vivo and in vitro, its molecular site of action remains to be determined. There has been, however, some preliminary study of newly discovered, specific gabapentin binding sites in neuronal tissues (see below).

Gabapentin appears to move across the gut and into the blood by a saturable transport mechanism competitively inhibited by L-leucine (Stewart et al., 1993) (the amino acid transporter known as system L). Experiments with the system L transport in cultured Chinese hamster ovary tumour cells also support the notion that gabapentin competes with leucine and is itself a substrate for transport by the system L. This may explain why gabapentin penetrates into the brain — the amino acid structure of gabapentin and the very high hydrophilicity of the compound would otherwise reduce its access across biological membranes. The time of peak anticonvulsant action with gabapentin is delayed about two hours after intravenous administration, past the time of peak drug concentration in either the blood plasma or the brain interstitial space (Welty *et al.*, 1993). These findings suggest that the anticonvulsant action of gabapentin may be due to delayed biochemical changes that require gabapentin to be present in neuronal cytoplasm, perhaps to interact with an intraneuronal enzyme or second drug receptor. Alternatively, gabapentin may require prolonged binding to an extracellular receptor before its anticonvulsant action become significant.

*In vitro*, gabapentin does not interact with neuronal sodium channels or L-type calcium channels (Taylor, 1993). Gabapentin is inactive at concentrations up to 100 μmol in standardized tests for interaction at $GABA_A$, $GABA_B$, benzodiazepine, glutamate, *N*-methyl-D-aspartate (NMDA), quisqualate, kainate, glycine, MK-801 and strychnine-insensitive glycine receptors. In addition many other neurotransmitter receptors have been screened, including A1 and A2 adenosine receptors; alpha-1, alpha-2 and beta adrenergic receptors; D1 and D2 dopamine receptors; histamine-1 receptors; S1 and S2 serotonin receptors; M1, M2 and nicotinic acetylcholine receptors; mu, delta, kappa and sigma opiate receptors; leukotriene $B_4$, $D_4$ and thromboxane $A_2$ receptors; phorbol ester dibutyrate receptors; and binding sites on calcium channels labelled by nifedipine and diltiazem and on sodium channels labelled by batrachotoxinin (Taylor, 1993). These negative results support the idea of a novel mechanism of anticonvulsant action for gabapentin.

## BINDING STUDIES AND RADIOLABELLED GABAPENTIN

Recent studies with $^3$H-gabapentin reveal a specific binding site in brain but not in other organs (Suman-Chauhan *et al.*, 1993). The gabapentin binding site is probably a protein, since specific binding activity is abolished by heating membranes to denaturing temperatures. It is likely to be membrane-bound because high levels of binding are seen in synaptosomal membrane fractions. The site is predominantly located on neurons, since binding is greatly reduced in striatal tissue pretreated *in vivo* with the selective neurotoxin ibotinic acid (Hill *et al.*, 1993).

Specific binding of gabapentin is highest in the superficial layers of neocortex and dendritic layers of hippocampus, with low levels of binding in white matter and brain stem (Hill *et al.*, 1993). Thus, gabapentin binding is most dense in areas rich in glutamatergic synapses, and the distribution is quite different from those of $GABA_A$, $GABA_B$ or dopamine receptors. The distribution of [3]H-gabapentin binding sites is somewhat different from those of NMDA-sensitive glutamate receptors. This is particularly true in the cerebellum, where [3]H-gabapentin sites are densest in the molecular layer but NMDA sites are densest in the granule cell layer (Naragos *et al.*, 1988). The distribution of [3]H-gabapentin binding sites bears a striking resemblance to those of [3]H-amino-3-hydroxy-5-methylisoxazole-4-propionic acid (AMPA) and [3]H-6-cyano-7-nitroquinoxaline-2-dione (CNQX) sites (Nielson *et al.*, 1990). AMPA is a selective agonist and CNQX is a selective antagonist for non-NMDA glutamate receptors involved in rapid excitatory synaptic transmission in the hippocampus, neocortex and other brain areas. However, the significance of the similarity in binding localization for [3]H-gabapentin and [3]H-AMPA is not clear, since the AMPA ligands quisqualate and L-glutamate have very low affinity for displacing [3]H-gabapentin binding (Suman-Chauhan *et al.*, 1993). In addition, gabapentin does not modulate excitatory postsynaptic potentials that depend on AMPA-type glutamate receptors.

Gabapentin binding is not affected by valproate, phenytoin, carbamazepine, phenobarbitone, diazepam, ethosuximide or many other neuroactive substances, in accordance with gabapentin's novel anticonvulsant pharmacology. However, gabapentin binding is displaced by L-leucine and various other system L amino acids ($IC_{50}$ values near 20 µM) (Thurlow *et al.*, 1993). The similarity and stereospecificity of these amino acids for displacement of [3]H-gabapentin binding and for system L transport *in vitro* indicates that the gabapentin binding site is closely associated with a component of the system L transport protein of brain cell membranes, and may represent a binding site on the transporter itself.

Gabapentin receptor binding is displaced by unlabelled gabapentin and by several structural analogues of gabapentin, including 3-isobutyl GABA. The two enantiomers of 3-isobutyl GABA have different potencies for binding at the gabapentin site, and the same difference in potency is seen in seizure models with whole animals (Taylor *et al.*, 1992). Several other compounds that are potent inhibitors of gabapentin binding *in vitro* also prevent seizures in animal models (Taylor *et al.*, 1992). Together, these findings strongly suggest that the gabapentin binding site is novel in comparison to commonly studied neurotransmitter and drug receptor sites of brain, and that the anticonvulsant actions of gabapentin and related compounds are correlated with binding at the gabapentin site, even though the physiological function of the binding site remains to be discovered.

Future biochemical studies may lead to the purification and identification of a protein receptor for gabapentin, such as a functionally characterized membrane-bound receptor, uptake transporter or enzyme.

# ANTICONVULSANT ACTIONS OF GABAPENTIN IN ANIMALS

Gabapentin prevents seizures induced by a wide variety of convulsant treatments in rodents and also prevents seizures in several genetic models. The results are summarized in Table 1. Effects in most models were seen from approximately half an hour after dosing to more than eight hours after dosing. The action of gabapentin in these animal models suggests that it may prevent generalized tonic–clonic seizures and partial seizures in clinical use.

**Table 1.**   Activity of gabapentin in animal models of seizures

| Species | Convulsive agent | Dose route | $ED_{50}$ (mg/kg) |
|---|---|---|---|
| Mouse | Tonic extensor seizure (maximal electroshock) | IP | 78 |
| Rat | Tonic extensor seizure (maximal electroshock) | PO | 9.1 |
| Rat | Tonic extensor seizure (maximal electroshock) | IV | 2.1 |
| Rat | Behavioural seizure score (hippocampal kindled rats) | IP | 30* |
| Mouse | Threshold clonic seizure (pentylenetetrazol) | IP | 47 |
| Mouse | Threshold clonic seizure (bicuculline) | IP | >500 |
| Mouse | Threshold clonic seizure (picrotoxin) | IP | >500 |
| Mouse | Threshold clonic seizure (strychnine) | IP | >500 |
| Mouse | Tonic extensor seizure (thiosemicarbazide) | IV | 6.3 |
| Mouse | Tonic extensor seizure (isoniazid) | PO | 20 |
| Mouse | Tonic extensor seizure (NMDA) | IP | >240† |
| Rat | Tonic extensor seizure (kainate) | IP | >300 |
| DBA/2J mouse | Tonic extensor seizure (audiogenic) | PO | 2.5 |
| Wistar rat | Absence seizure (EEG) (genetic predisposition) | IP | not effective (25–100 mg/kg) |
| Gerbil | Tonic extensor seizure (genetic predisposition) | PO | 15 |
| Gerbil | Clonic fore limb seizure (genetic predisposition) | PO | 19 |
| Baboon | Photogenic myoclonus (genetic predisposition) | IV | not effective (1.0–240 mg/kg) |

All results are from unpublished studies. IP, intraperitoneal; IV, intravenous; PO, oral.
*Lowest effective dose.
†At this dose, seizures were significantly delayed but not prevented.

Gabapentin prevents generalized convulsions in rodents that are genetically susceptible to seizures. However, non-convulsive absence-like seizures in rats are exacerbated by gabapentin. Results with a genetic model in baboons suggest that gabapentin is ineffective against photosensitive, myoclonic seizures. These results differentiate gabapentin from several other anticonvulsants that have different mechanisms of action.

Gabapentin is pharmacologically different from phenytoin, carbamazepine, lamotrigine and vigabatrin in that it prevents clonic seizures induced by the GABA antagonist pentylenetetrazol. Ethosuximide and valproic acid, agents that prevent absence seizures, also prevent pentylenetetrazol seizures. However, gabapentin did not prevent absence seizures in rats. Thus, there are significant differences between the anticonvulsant pharmacology of gabapentin and other anticonvulsant drugs, which again suggests that gabapentin has a novel anticonvulsant mechanism.

## CLINICAL PHARMACOKINETICS

The pharmacokinetic properties of gabapentin are summarized in Table 2.

In healthy volunteers, gabapentin is rapidly absorbed after oral administration. Maximum plasma levels occur two to three hours after administration and the elimination half-life ranges from five to seven hours (Vollmer et al., 1989). Gabapentin is not bound to plasma proteins and is not metabolized (Vollmer et al., 1986). It is excreted unchanged in the urine with renal clear-

**Table 2.**  Summary of gabapentin's pharmacokinetic properties

| Property | Clinical consequence |
|---|---|
| Maximum plasma concentration at 3 h | Satisfactory rate of absorption |
| No food effect | Dosing at any time |
| Repeated administration has no effect on pharmacokinetics | Multiple-dose kinetics; predictable single dose |
| Linear kinetics at therapeutic doses | Plasma concentration linearly related to dose |
| Limited absorption at high doses | Built-in protection against overdoses |
| No plasma protein binding | No interaction with other bound drugs |
| Not metabolized | Less interindividual variability in kinetics (in absence of renal disease) |
| Clearance linearly correlated with creatinine clearance | Adjustment of dose in renal failure can be based on creatinine clearance |
| Half-life of 5–7 h | Three daily doses probably necessary |

ance approximately equalling total clearance (120–130 ml/min). The renal clearance and elimination half-life are not altered by increasing dose, although oral bioavailability is reduced at higher doses. Gabapentin may be titrated to full therapeutic doses in two to three days with good tolerance. The pharmacokinetics of gabapentin are not altered following multiple dosing (Tuerck et al., 1989), and the bioavailability of gabapentin is not affected by food.

Gabapentin levels in a single specimen human brain were 80% of serum levels, confirming animal tissue distribution studies (Ojemann et al., 1988).

## DRUG INTERACTION STUDIES

A series of studies have been completed to detect possible interactions between gabapentin and other drugs. These have been either in patients receiving anticonvulsant monotherapy or in healthy subjects. An interaction between gabapentin and one of the established anticonvulsant drugs would influence the design and interpretation of phase 2 and 3 efficacy studies, and early evaluation of this possibility was important. Interactions in both directions have been sought, i.e. an effect of gabapentin on the kinetics of the established drugs and vice versa. In addition, selected potential interactions have been examined with the following compounds:

1. An aluminium/magnesium hydroxide antacid, because these preparations reduce the absorption of some drugs.
2. Cimetidine, which is a known inhibitor of the oxidative, drug-metabolizing system in the liver.
3. Probenecid, which can inhibit renal tubular secretion of acidic drugs.
4. The components of the combined oral contraceptive pill, the metabolism of which is enhanced by enzyme-inducing anticonvulsant drugs.

The conclusions reached as a result of these studies are summarized in Table 3. No detectable interaction occurs between gabapentin and the four anticonvulsants tested (Richens, 1992). This would be expected of a drug such as gabapentin, which is renally eliminated and not an inducer of hepatic microsomal enzymes.

The aluminium/magnesium antacid, Maalox TC, caused a slight reduction in the absorption of gabapentin, but no more than 20%, which is probably not of clinical significance (Busch et al., 1992). Surprisingly, cimetidine caused a 12% decrease in the renal clearance of gabapentin, but again this is unlikely to be of clinical importance. Probenecid, however, did not affect renal clearance, indicating that gabapentin does not undergo renal tubular secretion by the pathway that is blocked by probenecid. Finally, no effect of gabapentin was

**Table 3.**   Summary of drug interaction studies with gabapentin

| Drug | Effect of drug on gabapentin | Effect of gabapentin on drug |
|---|---|---|
| Phenytoin | None | None |
| Carbamazepine | None | None |
| Valproic acid | None | None |
| Phenobarbitone | None | None |
| Aluminium/magnesium hydroxide antacid (Maalox TC) | Slight reduced absorption | NT |
| Cimetidine | Slight reduced absorption | NT |
| Probenecid | None | NT |
| Norethynodrel | NT | None |
| Ethinyloestradiol | NT | None |

NT = not tested

seen on the kinetics of single doses of norethynodrel and ethinyloestradiol, which is predictive of a lack of interference with oral contraception.

Gabapentin's pharmacokinetic profile has many of the features of the ideal anticonvulsant drugs, and would be predicted to be a simple drug to use in clinical practice, in contrast to some of the currently available preparations.

## CLINICAL EFFICACY

After a 12-week baseline assessment with standard anticonvulsants, patients with partial seizures refractory to standard anticonvulsant drugs were randomly assigned to receive either placebo or gabapentin at doses of 600–1800 mg per day for 12 weeks, in three large, controlled studies (UK Gabapentin Study Group, 1990; Anhut et al., 1994; US Gabapentin Study Group, 1993). Gabapentin was given in addition to standard anticonvulsants and patient evaluation was performed in a double-blind fashion. Patients who completed double-blind treatment could continue gabapentin treatment as part of an open-label trial. All patients had partial (simple, complex or secondarily generalized) seizures refractory to marketed anticonvulsants, even though they were taking one or more drugs. Males and females 12 years of age or older were studied.

The primary efficacy criterion was reduction in the frequency of partial seizures from baseline to treatment levels. Seizure frequency was defined as the number of seizures per 28 days of observation. The primary efficacy parameters were response ratio (RR) and percentage change in frequency of seizures relative to the baseline.

The response ratio compares baseline seizure frequency ($B$) with treatment seizure frequency ($T$), as follows: $RR = (T - B)/(T + B)$. The response ratio avoids the skewing associated with percentage change and, since RR is normally distributed around zero, it allows parametric statistics to be used in the interpretation of the data. Values for RR range between $-1$ and $+1$. Negative values indicate a reduction (improvement) in seizure frequency during treatment, whereas positive values indicate an increase (worsening). An RR of $-0.33$ corresponds to a 50% reduction in seizure frequency relative to baseline seizure frequency.

A patient with at least a 50% reduction in partial seizure frequency (RR below $-0.33$) was classified as a responder. The percentage of patients who were responders is referred to as the responder rate.

Table 4 presents results for response ratio in placebo and gabapentin groups for the dosage specified prospectively by the trial protocol for efficacy comparison in each study. The mean RR was decreased (improved seizure control) in each study for patients who received gabapentin, compared with placebo. The difference between treatment groups was statistically significant in the intent-to-treat analysis in all studies.

Using combined data, the difference in mean response ratio between placebo and gabapentin treatment (gabapentin minus placebo) was calculated for each dosage level. Figure 1 presents these results, along with 95% confidence intervals. The estimated differences demonstrate a negative (improved) dose–effect progression and none of the ranges encompasses zero, indicating that gabapentin treatment results in dose-related seizure reduction in refractory patients. In addition, a linear regression of daily dose (mg per day) and RR was significant and gave a negative slope ($P = 0.0001$, $r^2 = 0.46$). At the

**Table 4.** Statistical comparisons of response ratio (RR) for efficacy dosages in three large, controlled studies

| Study/analysis | Efficacy dosage (mg/day) | Mean RR Placebo | Gabapentin | P |
|---|---|---|---|---|
| UK Study Group (1990) | 1200 | | | |
| Evaluable | | −0.060 | −0.192 | 0.0056 |
| Intent-to-treat | | −0.040 | −0.204 | 0.0018 |
| Anhut et al. (1994) | 1200 | | | |
| Evaluable | | −0.034 | −0.108 | 0.081 |
| Intent-to-treat | | −0.022 | −0.103 | 0.028 |
| US Study Group (1993) | 900 | | | |
| Evaluable | | −0.024 | −0.139 | 0.0038 |
| Intent-to-treat | | −0.017 | −0.138 | 0.0002 |

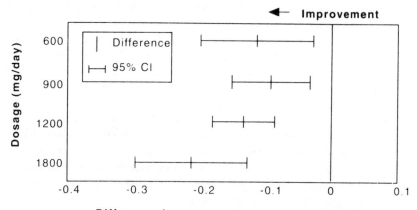

**Figure 1.** Difference in mean response ratio (gabapentin-placebo) and 95% confidence intervals: combined data from three large controlled studies (UK and US Gabapentin Study Groups (1990, 1993 respectively) and Anhut *et al*, 1994)

highest dose (1800 mg per day), gabapentin reduced total seizure frequency by 30% compared with placebo.

The analysis of responder rate also demonstrated improvement for patients who received gabapentin in each of the three controlled studies (Figure 2). In the analysis of combined data, responder rates were consistently higher for patients who received any dosage of gabapentin compared with those who received placebo, and a dose–response trend was evident. In the group of patients taking 1200 mg per day — which was the largest group and comparable in size to the placebo group — the responder rate was more than twice the rate seen in the placebo group.

The mean response ratio was analysed for all seizures and for four groups of partial seizures: simple partial, complex partial, partial seizures secondarily generalized, and partial seizures not secondarily generalized. The results for mean response ratio by seizure type for combined data from controlled studies (UK Gabapentin Study Group, 1990; US Gabapentin Study Group, 1993; Anhut *et al*, 1994) are presented in Figure 3.

The mean response ratio was consistently improved for all gabapentin treatment groups compared with placebo for all seizure types and for all seizures. Results indicate that gabapentin was particularly effective in patients with refractory complex partial seizures and partial seizures secondarily generalized.

**Long-term, open-label studies**

A total of 774 patients participated in five long-term, open-label studies. Patients were the same or were similar to those in the above double-blind

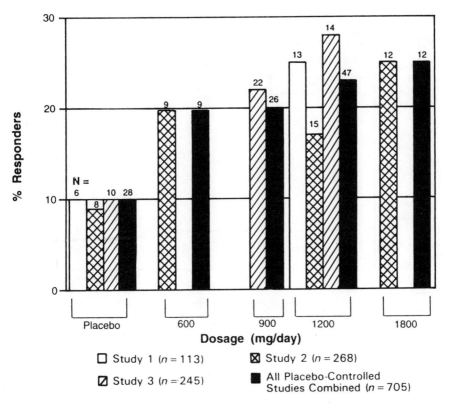

**Figure 2.** Responder rate in the three large controlled studies

studies. The majority of patients were receiving two concurrent anticonvulsants.

In two studies, in which all patients were initiating gabapentin therapy for the first time, the mean response ratio tended to decrease (improve) over time. The mean RR also improved over time in two of the open-label extensions of double-blind studies. Although improvement in the mean RR was not consistent over time, values remained within the range of −0.216 to −0.338 in all treatment periods. These results, which are displayed in Figure 4, indicate that the efficacy of gabapentin is maintained over time for these patient populations.

## SAFETY: CLINICAL STUDIES

By 1 January 1993 over 2000 people had been exposed to gabapentin. Of these, 448 healthy volunteers received the drug in pharmacokinetic studies.

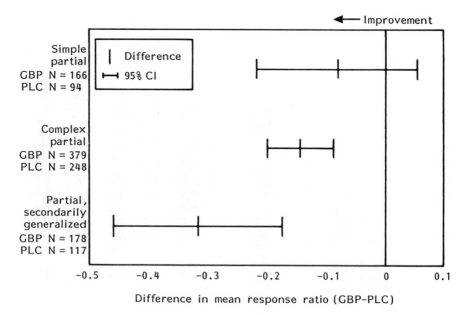

**Figure 3.**   Difference in mean response ratio

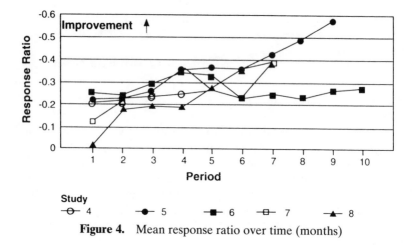

**Figure 4.**   Mean response ratio over time (months)

This number included 55 volunteers with renal disease and 52 volunteers with epilepsy. A total of 147 patients had taken gabapentin as monotherapy for conditions other than epilepsy (spasticity and migraine prophylaxis). Many patients have been treated long-term, with 657 patients receiving gabapentin for longer than one year, 376 for longer than two years, 219 for longer than three years and 116 for longer than four years. The longest any patient had received gabapentin was 7.3 years.

Gabapentin dosages up to 2400 mg per day were well tolerated despite being added to existing anticonvulsant therapy in refractory patients. No deaths were attributable to gabapentin and no serious adverse events were consistently attributable to gabapentin.

With short-term, add-on gabapentin therapy, there was an increased frequency of the types of adverse events that commonly occur with the use of currently marketed anticonvulsant drugs, particularly those symptoms related to the central nervous system and to the digestive system (Table 5). There was, however, no clear dose relationship for frequently occurring types of adverse events.

**Table 5.** Summary of the 10 adverse events occurring most frequently in patients receiving gabapentin

|  | Controlled studies | | All studies |
|---|---|---|---|
|  | Placebo $n = 307$ No. (%) | Gabapentin $n = 485$ No. (%) | Gabapentin $n = 1160$ No. (%) |
| Patients with more than one adverse event | 174 (56.7) | 369 (76.1) | 944 (81.4) |
| Adverse events: |  |  |  |
| Somnolence | 30 (9.8) | 98 (20.2) | 283 (24.4) |
| Dizziness | 24 (7.8) | 87 (17.9) | 235 (20.3) |
| Ataxia | 16 (5.2) | 64 (13.2) | 202 (17.4) |
| Fatigue | 15 (4.9) | 54 (11.1) | 171 (14.7) |
| Nystagmus | 15 (4.9) | 45 (9.3) | 174 (15.0) |
| Headache | 28 (9.1) | 42 (8.7) | 176 (15.2) |
| Tremor | 12 (3.9) | 35 (7.2) | 174 (15.0) |
| Diplopia | 6 (2.0) | 31 (6.4) | 124 (10.7) |
| Nausea and/or vomiting | 23 (7.5) | 29 (6.0) | 108 (9.3) |
| Rhinitis | 12 (3.0) | 22 (4.5) | 101 (8.7) |

Following initial therapy, long-term use of gabapentin at dosages of up to 2400 mg per day does not result in new or different adverse events or in increased frequency of adverse events in patients with epilepsy.

Unlike currently marketed anticonvulsant drugs, gabapentin has not been associated with liver injury, serious allergic reactions or changes in the haematopoietic system.

Clinical laboratory abnormalities have not been shown to change in association with gabapentin treatment.

## CONCLUSION

The treatment of patients with partial epilepsies remains a clinical problem and many people with these disorders remain refractory to increasing dosages of anticonvulsant drugs. Gabapentin is a drug of proved antiepileptic efficacy which is likely to be comparable with that of established compounds. Gabapentin treatment can be added to existing therapy relatively easily. The author's preference is to aim for an initial maintenance dose of 400 mg three times a day by administering increments of 400 mg at intervals of three or four days. Thereafter, depending on response, further increments to 800 mg three times daily can be given. Where a previously administered drug is being substituted with gabapentin, the latter can be introduced at a rate compatible with the withdrawal of the previous agent.

The advantages of gabapentin are likely to lie in its low potential for dose-related toxicity and drug hypersensitivity reactions. It has an almost ideal pharmacokinetic profile for an anticonvulsant: it is not metabolized, does not bind to plasma proteins, and does not appear to possess enzyme-inducing or inhibiting properties. There is no evidence of significant interaction with other anticonvulsants or with oral contraceptives. All of these observations imply that the drug should be simple to use in clinical practice and that plasma-level monitoring will not be required. Its only pharmacokinetic defect is its relatively short half-life. Existing studies tested efficacy with dosing three times daily, which is a less than ideal regimen for the treatment of epilepsy. Studies of efficacy with twice-daily dosing will be important.

Gabapentin appears to show a low relative toxicity for a potential anticonvulsant drug, as shown by the mild nature of complaints in clinical trials and the high retention rate within studies. The advantages of gabapentin over other drugs in this area are difficult to assess, and there is a need to develop standardized tools for evaluating dose-related central nervous system effects of anticonvulsant drugs, as well as evaluating their cost–benefit ratios.

The efficacy of gabapentin in partial seizures warrants further evaluation in a number of areas. In the future, the efficacy of monotherapy using this drug may be demonstrated. Studies of previously untreated patients could be started in which gabapentin would be used over longer periods of time and its efficacy established relative to currently available anticonvulsants. Because 70% of patients presenting with epilepsy for the first time respond rapidly to low doses of anticonvulsant drugs by attaining remission (Annegers et al., 1979), drugs such as gabapentin may have particular value in such a population. There is a need to define the spectrum of activity of gabapentin in further controlled studies. Efficacy is currently only proved against partial seizures, but a variety of generalized seizures (particularly in children) remain a clinical problem, with existing drugs often providing inadequate control. Again, the lack of dose-related central nervous system effects with gabapentin may be particularly important in children with epilepsy, in whom cognitive function, learning and behaviour are important considerations. Thus, children with epilepsy may benefit from the further study of gabapentin in paediatric populations.

## ACKNOWLEDGEMENT

I am grateful to Dr Charles Taylor for his help in the preparation of this review and to all those colleagues who collaborated in clinical studies.

## REFERENCES

Anhut H, Ashman P, Feuerstein TJ et al. (1993) Gabapentin as add-on therapy in patients with partial seizures: a double-blind, placebo-controlled study. Epilepsia (in press).

Annegers JF, Hauser WA and Elverback LR (1979) Remission of seizures and relapse in patients with epilepsy. Epilepsia, 20, 729–737.

Bartoszyk GD, Meyerson N, Peimann W (1986) In: Current Problems in Epilepsy 4. New Antiepileptic Drugs (eds. BS Meldrum and RJ Porter), pp 147–163, Libbey, London.

Busch JA, Radulovic LL, Bockbrader HN, Underwood BA, Sedman AJ and Chang T (1992) Effect of Maalox TC on single-dose pharmacokinetics of gabapentin capsules in healthy subjects. Pharm. Res., 9 (suppl. 10), S315.

Hengy H and Kolle E (1985) Determination of gabapentin in plasma and urine by high-performance liquid chromatography and pre-column labelling for ultraviolet detection. J. Chromatogr., 341, 473–478.

Hill DR, Suman-Chauhan N and Woodruff GN (1993) Localisation of [³H]-gabapentin to a novel site in rat brain: autoradiographic studies. Eur. J. Pharmacol., 224, 303–309.

Loscher W., Honack D and Taylor CP (1991) Gabapentin increases amino-oxyacetic acid-induced GABA accumulation in several regions of rat brain. Neurosci. Lett., 128, 150–154.

Naragos WF, Penney JB and Young AB (1988) Anatomic correlation of NMDA and [³H]-TCP-labelled receptors in rat brain. J. Neurosci., 8, 493–501.

Nielson EO, Drejer J, Cha J-HJ, Young AB and Honore T (1990) Autoradiographic characterization and localization of quisqualate binding sites in rat brain using the antagonist [³H]6-cyano-7-nitroquinoxaline-2,3-dione: comparison with (r,S)–[³H]alpha-amino-3-hydroxy-5-methyl-4-isoxazoleproprionic acid binding sites. J. Neurochem., 54, 686–695.

Ojemann LM, Friel PN and Ojemann GA (1988) Gabapentin concentrations in human brain. Epilepsia, 29, 694.

Richens A (1993) Clinical pharmacokinetics of gabapentin. In: New Trends in Epilepsy Management: The Role of Gabapentin (ed. D Chadwick), International Congress and Symposium Series No. 198, pp. 41–46. Royal Society of Medicine, London.

Stewart BH, Kugler AR, Thompson PR and Bockbrader HN (1993) A saturable transport mechanism in the intestinal absorption of gabapentin is the underlying cause of the lack of proportionality between increasing dose and drug levels in plasma. *Pharm. Res.*, **10**, 276-281.

Suman-Chauhan N, Webdale L, Hill DR and Woodruff GN (1993) Characterisation of [³H]gabapentin binding to a novel site in rat brain: homogenate binding studies. *Eur. J. Pharmacol.*, **244**, 293–301.

Taylor CP (1993) Mechanism of action of new antiepileptic drugs. In: *New Trends in Epilepsy: The Role of Gabapentin* (ed. D Chadwick), International Congres and Symposium Series No. 198. Royal Society of Medicine, London.

Taylor CP, Vartanian MG, Yuen P-W, Bigge C, Suman-Chauhan N and Hill DR (1992) Potent and stereospecific anticonvulsant activity of 3-isobutyl GABA related to in vitro binding at a novel site labelled by titrated gabapentin. *Epilepsy Res.*, **14**, 11–15.

Thurlow RJ, Brown JP, Gee NS, Hill DR and Woodruff GN (1993) [³H]-gabapentin may label a system-L like neutral amino acid carrier in brain. *Eur. J. Pharmacol.*, **247**, 3441–3445.

Tuerck D, Vollmer K, Bockbrader H and Sedman A (1989) Dose-linearity of the new anticonvulsant gabapentin after multiple oral doses. *Eur. J. Clin. Pharmacol.*, **36** (suppl. A310).

UK Gabapentin Study Group (1990) Gabapentin in partial epilepsy. *Lancet*, **i**, 1114–1117.

US Gabapentin Study Group (1993) Gabapentin as add-on therapy in refractory epilepsy: a double-blind, placebo-controlled, parallel-group study. *Neurology*, **43**, 2292–2298.

Vollmer K, Anhut H, Thomann P (1989) Pharmacokinetic model and absolute bio-availability of the new anticonvulsant gabapentin. *Adv. Epileptology*, **17**, 209–211.

Vollmer K, von Hodenberg A and Kolle E (1986) Pharmacokinetics and metabolism of gabapentin in rat, dog and man. *Drug Res.*, **36**, 830–839.

Welty DF, Schielke GP, Vartanian MG and Taylor CP (1993) Gabapentin anticonvulsant action in rats: disequilibrium with peak drug concentration in plasma and brain microdialysate. *Epilepsy Res.*, **16**, 175–181.

# 6

# Lamotrigine

Ilo E. Leppik
*University of Minnesota, and MINCEP Epilepsy Care, USA*

## INTRODUCTION

Lamotrigine is one of the new anticonvulsant medications which appears to have great promise in clinical use (Graves and Leppik, 1991). Observations that folates could produce seizures in animals and that anticonvulsant drugs could lead to an impairment of folate metabolism led to the screening of antifolates for anticonvulsant activity (Rogawski and Porter, 1990; Yuen, 1991). Lamotrigine, a phenyltriazine, emerged from this programme. Its chemical name is 3,5-diamino-6-(2,3-dichlorophenyl)-1,2,4-triazine, and it is structurally and chemically unrelated to other anticonvulsant drugs. It has a molecular weight of 256, a $pK_a$ of 5.5 and relatively low water solubility, approximately 0.17 g/l.

A number of assays have been developed to measure lamotrigine concentration in biological fluids. Some of the earlier ones involved high-pressure liquid chromatography (HPLC) (Cohen *et al.*, 1987). A more recently developed HPLC assay is more rapid and has a sensitivity limit of 0.1 mg/l (Fazio *et al.*, 1992). One assay can measure lamotrigine and its major metabolite simultaneously (Sinz and Remmel, 1991). A radioimmunoassay sensitive to 20 ng/ml (Biddlecombe *et al.*, 1990) and an immunofluorometric assay (Sailstad and Findlay, 1991) are available and may become useful in clinical settings. Approximately 55% of the total lamotrigine measured is protein-bound, and valproate does not affect plasma protein binding of lamotrigine (Trnavska *et al.*, 1991).

## MECHANISM OF ACTION

Although its precise mechanism of action remains to be determined, lamotrigine most probably exerts its anticonvulsant activity by inhibiting the

---

*New Anticonvulsants: Advances in the Treatment of Epilepsy.* Edited by M. R. Trimble release of excitatory amino acids (Lamb *et al.*, 1985; Leach *et al.*, 1986). Lamotrigine inhibits veratrine-evoked release of endogenous glutamate, and also blocks aspartate release but only at high veratrine concentrations.

A recent study of voltage-sensitive sodium channels shows that lamotrigine inhibits sodium channels in a similar manner to phenytoin and carbamazepine (Lang *et al.*, 1993). In another study, lamotrigine was found to block sustained repetitive firing of sodium-dependent action potentials in mouse spinal cord cultured neurons and inhibit [3H]batrachotoxinin. This study also demonstrated binding in rat brain synaptosomes, suggesting a direct interaction with voltage-activated sodium channels (Cheung *et al.*, 1992). Unitary, fast, presumptive-sodium spikes, evoked at low frequencies, were not blocked significantly by lamotrigine. In contrast, burst firing induced by pulsed application of L-glutamate or potassium ions was markedly depressed at 10 μM. Presumptive calcium currents were inhibited by lamotrigine at 100 μM. It is proposed that the drug inhibits epileptiform burst firing preferentially by state or activity-dependent interactions with voltage-gated cation channels, principally the sodium channel (Lees and Leach, 1993). Even though it is structurally related to antifolate drugs, this drug has only very weak activity against folate in animal models.

## PRECLINICAL EFFICACY AND SAFETY

Anticonvulsant properties of lamotrigine have been evaluated in a number of animal models. The anticonvulsant profile following oral administration in two standard anticonvulsant tests, the maximal electroshock test in mice and rats and the pentylenetetrazol infusion test in mice, was studied in comparison with the known anticonvulsant drugs phenytoin, phenobarbitone, diazepam, carbamazepine, valproate and ethosuximide. In the maximal electroshock test, of the drugs examined, lamotrigine was ranked the most potent and persistent in both species. Clonus latency in the pentylenetetrazol test was not increased by lamotrigine, phenytoin or carbamazepine, but was significantly increased by the remaining anticonvulsants. Thus, lamotrigine resembled phenytoin and carbamazepine in its ability to block hind-limb extension induced by maximal electroshock, but not to increase pentylenetetrazol-induced clonus latency (Miller *et al.*, 1986). These results suggest that lamotrigine may be of value in the treatment of generalized tonic–clonic and partial seizures.

Lamotrigine is also effective against sound-induced seizures in genetically epilepsy-prone rats, and though more potent than phenytoin in this model, it was less effective than compounds that decrease glutamatergic neurotransmission, including excitatory amino acid antagonists acting at *N*-methyl-D-aspartate (NMDA) receptors (Smith *et al.*, 1993a).

Acute dosage behavioural studies in mice and rats have shown a wide separation between anticonvulsant doses and doses producing behavioural impairment (Miller et al., 1986). In a test of working memory and phencyclidine discrimination studies, lamotrigine did not impair working memory in rats at doses that caused temporary sedation and ataxia (Leach et al., 1991). In the gerbil model of global ischaemia, high doses of lamotrigine provided protection against damage to the CA-1 region of the hippocampus (Leach et al., 1991).

There is a wide gap between the effective and lethal doses in rodent species. The median effective dose of lamotrigine in the maximal electroshock test was 2–4 mg/kg. In contrast, the median dose at which half the animals died was 160–250 mg/kg. Chronic toxicity studies in rodents and primates at doses of up to 20–125 mg/kg per day have shown no toxic effects on organ systems or laboratory determinations (Miller et al., 1986). Lamotrigine has not shown teratogenic effects in reproductive studies in animals. These results indicate the potential for relatively low toxicity in humans.

## METABOLISM

Lamotrigine undergoes glucuronidation on the 2-nitrogen atom of the triazine ring, leading to a quaternary ammonium-linked glucuronide in humans and animals (Sinz and Remmel, 1991; Magdalou et al., 1992). This reaction proceeds with an apparent $V_{max}$ of 0.65 nmol/min.mg and $K_m$ of 2.56 mM in human hepatocytes. The average value of lamotrigine glucuronidation in four human samples of transplantable liver was 0.43± 0.14 nmol/min.mg, indicating the possibility of a large interindividual variation in a patient population. Among the drugs that undergo quaternary ammonium-linked glucuronidation, chlorpromazine — but not imipramine, amitriptyline and cyproheptadine — inhibited the glucuronidation of lamotrigine in vitro (Magdalou et al., 1992).

In human volunteers, concomitant administration of sodium valproate reduced total clearance of lamotrigine and significantly increased elimination half-life. Reduced clearance of lamotrigine occurred within the first hour but renal elimination was not impaired. This strongly suggests that hepatic competition between valproate and lamotrigine for glucuronidation occurs (Yuen et al., 1992). In a study of the effect of a genetic deficit in glucuronidation on lamotrigine metabolism, a single oral dose of the drug was administered to seven volunteers with Gilbert's syndrome (unconjugated hyperbilirubinaemia). In these subjects mean oral clearance was 32% lower ($P < 0.01$) and the plasma elimination half-life ($t_{1/2}$) was 37% lower ($P < 0.02$) than in the normal controls. The amount of unchanged drug excreted in the urine was 30% greater in the Gilbert's syndrome subjects (Posner et al., 1989). The lamotrigine glucuronide is then almost completely excreted by the kidneys.

## PHARMACOKINETICS

Absorption of lamotrigine is rapid; in 10 subjects without epilepsy a single oral dose of 120 mg had a time to peak concentration ($T_{max}$) of 2.75 ± 1.29 hours, with the maximum concentration ($C_{max}$) of 1.6 ± 0.33 mg/l and a volume of distribution ($Vd$) of 1.1 l/kg (Table 1). Doses of 240 mg in volunteers were associated with peak concentrations of approximately 3 mg/l (Peck, 1991). The drug's elimination half-life in these subjects was 24.1 ± 5.7 hours (Cohen et al., 1984). In a multiple-dose study of 10 volunteers receiving lamotrigine for seven days, $t_{1/2}$ was 25.5 ± 10.2 hours, suggesting no autoinduction of metabolism over this short time (Cohen et al., 1987). In a study of patients receiving other anticonvulsant drugs, the half-life of lamotrigine was decreased to 14.6 ± 6.9 hours in patients receiving liver enzyme-inducing anticonvulsant drugs. In patients receiving valproate along with inducers the half-life was similar to that in normal volunteers, 29.6 ± 10 hours (Jawad et al., 1987). Valproate increases lamotrigine's half-life, to a mean of 59 hours, with a range of 30.5 hours to 88.8 hours (Binnie et al., 1986). Recent clinical experience has shown that felbamate also increases the half-life of lamotrigine, probably to the same degree as valproate. The plasma concentrations of co-administered valproate, phenytoin, carbamazepine, phenobarbitone and primidone were not altered by lamotrigine (Jawad et al., 1987). Lamotrigine follows linear kinetics (Ramsay et al., 1991). A study of four patients receiving lamotrigine for up to 104 weeks showed drug clearances (dose/area under curve) of 0.0436 ± 0.0171, 0.0468 ± 0.0093 and 0.0575 ± 0.0160 l/h.kg on days 63, 70 and 133, indicating that it does not induce its own metabolism (Mikati et al., 1989).

**Table 1.**   Characteristics of lamotrigine

| | |
|---|---|
| Molecular weight | 256 |
| $pK_a$ | 5.5 |
| Protein binding | 55% |
| Absorption | 2–4 hours |
| Volume of distribution | 1.1 l/kg |
| Half-life: | |
|     volunteers | 24 hours |
|     patients on inducers | 14 hours |
|     patients on inducers plus inhibitors | 24 hours |
|     paitnets on inhibitors | 60 hours |
| Elimination kinetics | Linear |
| Effective blood levels | 2–4 mg/l* |
| Daily doses: | |
|     patients on inducers | 400–600 mg/day* |
|     patients on inhibitors | 200–300 mg/day* |

*Subject to change with more experience.

An interaction between lamotrigine and carbamazepine 10,11-epoxide has been observed. In nine consecutive patients the mean serum carbamazepine 10,11-epoxide concentration increased by 45% ($P < 0.01$) and the ratio of carbamazepine 10,11-epoxide to carbamazepine increased by 19% ($P < 0.02$). In four patients these changes were associated with dizziness, nausea and diplopia (Warner et al., 1992).

In a double-blind, randomized, cross-over, placebo-controlled study, the effect of multiple oral doses of paracetamol on lamotrigine disposition was examined in healthy volunteers. Area under the plasma concentration–time curve for lamotrigine decreased by 20% ($P > 0.01$), and the half-life decreased by 15% ($P > 0.01$) when the drug was concurrently administered with paracetamol (Depot et al., 1990).

## CLINICAL EFFICACY

Early, limited studies were encouraging. An open study of 20 patients given doses of 50 mg per day to 225 mg twice a day for one week showed that there were significantly fewer seizures ($P > 0.01$) during treatment compared with baseline frequency (Jawad et al., 1987). In a double-blind, placebo-controlled, cross-over add-on study of 10 patients receiving 100–300 mg per day lamotrigine for one week, six patients had a 50% or greater reduction in seizures (Binnie et al., 1987).

A number of double-blind, placebo-controlled studies of lamotrigine in refractory epilepsy have been completed (Table 2). In the study carried out in the Netherlands, 30 patients completed a cross-over study with two treatment periods of three months separated by a six-week cross-over period. The median reduction of seizures was 17%, significant with a value of $P > 0.02$ (Binnie et al., 1989). A cross-over study of 20 adult patients in Wales using 12-week treatment periods and lamotrigine doses of 75–400 mg per day showed a median reduction in total seizures of 59% (Jawad et al., 1989). One study with 18 completed patients performed at the Chalfont Centre, UK, also using a 12-week study period with a six-week cross-over, did not show a difference between placebo and lamotrigine over the whole study period, although a 'marked reduction' in generalized tonic–clonic seizures was observed in the last four weeks of lamotrigine treatment (Sander et al., 1990a). A study from France evaluated 23 adult patients over a two-month treatment period. Seven patients had a greater than 50% reduction in overall seizure frequency (Loiseau et al., 1990).

A multicentre, double-blind, cross-over study with 14-week treatment periods was carried out in the USA. Eighty-eight patients completed the protocol, with the majority (69) receiving 400 mg of lamotrigine. Mean trough plasma concentrations ranged from 1.64 mg/l to 2.94 mg/l. The median

**Table 2.**  Summary of reported double-blind, placebo-controlled, add-on trials of lamotrigine

| No. of patients | Median reduction of all seizures* (%) | Probability values | | | References |
| | | Total seizures | Partial seizures | Generalized seizures | |
| --- | --- | --- | --- | --- | --- |
| 30 | 17 | > 0.02 | > 0.01 | NA | Binnie et al. (1989) |
| 21 | 59 | > 0.002 | > 0.001 | > 0.05 | Jawad et al. (1989) |
| 18 | 18 | NS | NS | > 0.05† | Sander et al. (1990b) |
| 23 | 23 | > 0.05 | > 0.05 | NA | Loiseau et al (1990) |
| 88 | 25 | > 0.001 | – | – | Risner et al. (1990) |
| 41 | – | > 0.0001 | > 0.05 | NS | Schapel et al. (1993) |
| 59** | 36 | – | > 0.007 | – | Matsuo et al. (1993) |

*Partial seizures plus generalized tonic–clonic seizures.
†Analysis of last 8 weeks of treatment.
NA, not applicable; NS, not significant.
**500mg lamotrigine.

reduction in seizure frequency was 25% ($P > 0.001$ compared with placebo), and 20% of patients had a 50% or greater reduction (Rinser et al., 1990).

A study from Australia involved 41 patients in a cross-over study with 12-week observation periods. Doses of lamotrigine were 150 mg or 300 mg per day, designed to achieve plasma levels of 1–3 mg/l. There was a highly significant ($P > 0.001$) decrease in total seizure counts (Schapel et al., 1993).

A recent study of 81 patients aged 15–67 years, using a cross-over design with 18-week study periods, used both seizure frequency and a health-related quality of life (HRQL) assessment to measure outcome. The mean reduction of all seizure types relative to placebo was 29% ($P > 0.0001$) and 11 experienced a greater than 50% reduction in total seizures (Smith et al., 1993b). The HRQL also showed statistically significant improvement over placebo in two of the scales; happiness ($P = 0.003$) and mastery ($P = 0.003$).

In addition to the controlled studies, lamotrigine has been administered to over 2000 65 patients in settings that have allowed safety and efficacy data to be collected (Richens and Yuen, 1991). A large number of these trials have been open add-on studies, and data from 27 of them, comprising 572 patients, have been pooled in Table 3 to attempt to obtain some indication of the spectrum of lamotrigine activity (Richens and Yuen, 1991). These preliminary observations indicate that lamotrigine may have activity against a number of seizure types in adults as well as children. Two reports of lamotrigine in Lennox–Gastaut syndrome have been favourable (Timmings and Richens, 1992; Schlumberger et al., 1994). Absence epilepsy has also responded favourably. There has been one report of status epilepticus being treated with a 600 mg dose of lamotrigine given by nasogastric tube over four hours (Pisani et al., 1989) after diazepam failed.

**Table 3.** Percentage of patients with a 50% or greater reduction in seizures in the first 12 weeks of lamotrigine treatment. Data pooled from 27 open add-on studies involving 572 patients

| Seizure type | % | Total patients |
|---|---|---|
| All | 30 | 417 |
| Partial | 28 | 308 |
| Tonic–clonic | 52 | 209 |
| Absence | 46 | 24 |
| Atypical absence | 64 | 11 |
| Myoclonic | 36 | 11 |
| Atonic | 50 | 14 |

Data from Richens and Yuen (1991).

In addition to evaluating seizures, a number of studies have also examined the effect of lamotrigine on electroencephalographic (EEG) activity (Van Wieringen et al., 1987). In one study of 16 subjects, five patients who had frequent interictal spike activity had a reduction of 78–98% in discharges following a single oral dose of 120 mg or 240 mg lamotrigine (Binnie et al., 1986). All six patients with photosensitivity showed a marked reduction to photic stimulation, with the response being abolished in two patients (Binnie et al., 1986). Another study of interictal spike counts involved a three-way cross-over with placebo, diazepam 20 mg and lamotrigine 240 mg in six patients. Both treatments significantly reduced interictal spikes as compared with placebo (Jawad et al., 1986). However, a subsequent survey has shown that the EEG may be of doubtful value as an outcome variable in clinical anticonvulsant drug trials in general, although positive correlations have been noted for lamotrigine (Van Wieringen et al., 1989).

In addition to the drug's use in epilepsy, one report describes five patients with Parkinson's disease who showed some positive effects from treatment with lamotrigine (Zipp et al., 1993).

## ADVERSE EFFECTS

Lamotrigine is generally well tolerated. The most often reported adverse effects may be dose-related and are most commonly observed in patients receiving more than one additional anticonvulsant medication. These adverse effects include diplopia, drowsiness, dizziness, ataxia, headache, nausea and vomiting (Binnie *et al.*, 1988, 1989; Jawad *et al.*, 1989; Loiseau *et al.*, 1990; Risner *et al.*, 1990; Sander *et al.*, 1990; Richens and Yuen, 1991; Smith *et al.*, 1993b).

One meta-analysis of the clinical safety of lamotrigine evaluated four randomized, double-blind, placebo-controlled, cross-over trials in which this drug was added to existing anticonvulsant therapy of 92 adult patients with refractory epilepsy. Although higher, the incidence of adverse experiences with lamotrigine did not differ significantly from placebo (Betts *et al.*, 1991). In an analysis of 27 open studies with 12-month treatment periods, pooled data from 572 patients indicated that the most commonly reported adverse experiences were dizziness, diplopia, somnolence, headache, ataxia and asthenia (10–14% incidence). Forty-nine patients (8.6%) were withdrawn because of adverse events, usually consisting of an inability to tolerate the drug because of unpleasant symptoms. The single most common reason for discontinuation was rash, which occurred in 2.3% of the subjects (Betts *et al.*, 1991). Most rashes began within two weeks of initiation of lamotrigine and resolved within days of discontinuation (Betts *et al.*, 1991).

Neuropsychological function has been evaluated in 10 adult subjects. Although statistical analysis proved impracticable due to differing scores across cells, there appeared to be a marginal reduction in 'general cerebral efficiency' during the lamotrigine phase compared with placebo (Banks and Beran, 1991). Further studies are indicated to define more clearly what effect, if any, lamotrigine has on cognitive functioning.

Biochemical and haematological parameters are unaltered by lamotrigine therapy. The effect of this drug on serum folate and red cell folate concentrations was assessed in a series of 14 patients treated for up to five years. These patients showed no significant difference in red cell folate concentrations after chronic treatment compared with levels prior to therapy (Sander and Patsalos, 1992).

## CLINICAL USE

The initial dose of lamotrigine in adults depends on what other anticonvulsant drug the patient is taking. In patients taking enzyme-inducing anticonvulsants such as carbamazepine, phenytoin and phenobarbitone, lamotrigine should be started at a dose of 50 mg twice daily, and after two weeks increased to 100 mg twice daily; after an additional two weeks the dose can be increased to 100 mg three times daily. After a dose of 300 mg per day is reached, the dose should be increased gradually, at increments of 50 mg every two weeks, until seizures are controlled or dose-related side-effects occur. Most patients respond to doses of 400 mg per day, but doses above 600–700 mg per day may provide additional seizure control. Dose-related side-effects, especially nausea, unsteadiness, dizziness and ataxia are more common when lamotrigine is used in combination with carbamazepine and phenytoin. In patients who are taking anticonvulsant drugs that are inducers (phenytoin, carbamazepine, phenobarbitone) as well as inhibitors of lamotrigine metabolism (valproate) the dose may be started and increased as described above. However, the total daily dose usually cannot be increased above 300 mg without significant side-effects. If adverse effects develop, withdrawal of valproate should be considered.

Because valproate inhibits the elimination of lamotrigine, in patients on valproate monotherapy the initial dose and subsequent increments should be made more gradually. A recommended starting dose is 25 mg twice daily, increasing by 25 mg per day increments at two-week intervals, with close monitoring for side-effects, which are common when the dose is higher than 200 mg per day. Seizure control is unlikely to improve with lamotrigine doses over 300 mg per day in patients also taking valproate. If the valproate dosage is subsequently tapered off or discontinued, the lamotrigine dose may need to be increased, and will probably be better tolerated.

## CONCLUSION

Lamotrigine appears to be a useful addition to the present group of drugs for the treatment of epilepsy. It has been most widely studied as add-on therapy in patients with intractable partial seizures, and has been found to be effective in these patients. Its spectrum may be wider than controlled trials indicate, and it has been successful in the Lennox–Gastaut syndrome and absence seizures. Its potency in clinical studies is comparable to that of most of the other new drugs. No direct comparisons of efficacy have been performed. Lamotrigine may be useful as monotherapy, but experience is limited. It has few side-effects, and some reports suggest it may even have some positive effects. It does not affect folate concentrations or other laboratory parameters. It has a moderately long half-life which is greatly influenced by other medications. Because no association has been found with animal teratogenesis, it is potentially useful in women of childbearing age. In March 1993 the US Food and Drug Administration scientific advisory panel recommended approval in the USA for lamotrigine as treatment for adults with partial and secondary generalized seizures. Lamotrigine is available in most European countries.

## REFERENCES

Banks GK and Beran RG (1991) Neuropsychological assessment in lamotrigine treated epileptic patients. *Clin. Exp. Neurol.*, **28**, 230–237.

Betts T, Goodwin G, Withers RM and Yuen AW (1991) Human safety of lamotrigine. *Epilepsia*, **32** (suppl. 2), S17–21.

Biddlecombe RA, Dean KL, Smith CD and Jeal SC (1990) Validation of a radioimmunoassay for the determination of human plasma concentrations of lamotrigine. *J. Pharm. Biomed. Anal.*, **8** (8–12), 691–694.

Binnie CD, van Emde Boas W, Kasteleijn-Nolste-Trenite DG *et al.* (1986) Acute effects of lamotrigine (BW430C) in persons with epilepsy. *Epilepsia*, **27**(3), 248–54.

Binnie CD, Beintema DJ, Debets RM *et al.* (1987) Seven day administration of lamotrigine in epilepsy: placebo-controlled add-on trial. *Epilepsy Res.*, **1**(3), 202–208.

Binnie CD (1988) Preliminary evaluation of potential anti-epileptic drugs by single dose electrophysiological and pharmacological studies in patients. *J. Neural. Transm.*, **72** (3), 259–266.

Binnie CD, Debets RM, Engelsman M *et al.* (1989) Double-blind crossover trial of lamotrigine (Lamictal) as add-on therapy in intractable epilepsy. *Epilepsy Res.*, **4** (3), 222–229.

Cheung H, Kamp D and Harris E (1992) An in vitro investigation of the action of lamotrigine on neuronal voltage-activated sodium channels. *Epilepsy Res.*, **13** (2), 107–112.

Cohen AF, Fowle ASE, Land GS and Bye A (1984) BW340C — A new anticonvulsant. Pharmacokinetics in normal man. *Epilepsia*, **25**, 656.

Cohen AF, Land GS, Breimer DD, Yuen WC, Winton C and Peck AW (1987) Lamotrigine, a new anticonvulsant: pharmacokinetics in normal humans. *Clin. Pharmacol. Therap.*, **42**, 535–541.

Depot M, Powell JR, Messenheimer JA Jr, Cloutier G and Dalton MJ (1990) Kinetic effects of multiple oral doses of acetaminophen on a single oral dose of lamotrigine. *Clin. Pharmacol. Therap.*, **48** (4), 346–355.

Fazio A, Artesi C, Russo M, Trio R, Oteri G and Pisani F (1992) A liquid chromatographic assay using a high-speed column for the determination of lamotrigine, a new antiepileptic drug, in human plasma. *Ther. Drug Monit.*, **14** (6), 509–512.

Graves NM and Leppik IE (1991) Antiepileptic medications in development. *DICP Ann. Pharmacother.*, **25**, 978–986.

Jawad S, Oxley J, Yuen WC and Richens A (1986) The effect of lamotrigine, a novel anticonvulsant, on interictal spikes in patients with epilepsy. *Br. J. Clin. Pharmacol.*, **22** (2), 191–93.

Jawad S, Yuen WC, Peck AW, Hamilton MJ, Oxley JR and Richens A (1987) Lamotrigine: single-dose pharmacokinetics and initial 1 week experience in refractory epilepsy. *Epilepsy Res.*, **1** (3), 194–201.

Jawad S, Richens A, Goodwin G and Yuen WC (1989) Controlled trial of lamotrigine (Lamictal) for refractory partial seizures. *Epilepsia*, **30** (3), 356–363.

Lang DG, Wang CM and Cooper BR (1993) Lamotrigine, phenytoin and carbamazepine interactions on the sodium current present in N4TG1 mouse neuroblastoma cells. *J. Pharmacol. Exp. Ther.*, **266** (2), 829–835.

Lamb RJ, Leach MJ, Miller AA and Wheatley PL (1985) Anticonvulsant profile in mice of lamotrigine, a novel anticonvulsant. *Br. J. Pharmacol.*, **85**, 366P.

Leach MJ, Marden CM and Miller AA (1986) Pharmacological studies on lamotrigine, a novel potential antiepileptic drug: II. Neurochemical studies on the mechanism of action. *Epilepsia*, **27** (5), 490–497.

Leach MJ, Baxter MG and Critchley MAE (1991) Neurochemical and behavioral aspects of lamotrigine. *Epilepsia*, **32** (suppl. 2), S4–S8.

Lees G and Leach MJ (1993) Studies on the mechanism of action of the novel anticonvulsant lamotrigine (Lamictal) using primary neurological cultures from rat cortex. *Brain Res.*, **612** (1–2), 190–199.

Loiseau P, Yuen AW, Duche B, Menager T and Arne-Bes MC (1990) A randomised double-blind placebo-controlled crossover add-on trial of lamotrigine in patients with treatment-resistant partial seizures. *Epilepsy Res.*, **7** (2), 136–145.

Magdalou J, Herber R, Bidault R and Siest G (1992) In vitro N-glucuronidation of a novel antiepileptic drug, lamotrigine, by human liver microsomnes. *J. Pharmacol. Exp. Ther.*, **260** (3), 1166–1173.

Matsuo F, Bergen D, Faught E, Messenheimer JA, Dren AT, Rudd GD and Lineberry CG (1993) Placebo-controlled study of the efficacy and safety of lamotrigine in patients with partial seizures. *Neurology*, **43**, 2284–2291.

Mikati MA, Schachter SC, Schomer DL et al. (1989) Long-term tolerability, pharmacokinetic and preliminary efficacy study of lamotrigine in patients with resistant partial seizures. *Clin. Neuropharmacol.*, **12** (4), 312–321.

Miller AA, Wheatley P, Sawyer DA, Baxter MG and Roth B (1986) Pharmacological studies on lamotrigine, a novel potential antiepileptic drug: I. Anticonvulsant profile in mice and rats. *Epilepsia*, **27** (5), 483–489.

Peck AW (1991) Clinical pharmacology of lamotrigine. *Epilepsia*, **32** (suppl. 2), S9–12.

Pisani F, Gallitto G and Di Perri RJ (1991) Could lamotrigine be useful in status epilepticus? A case report (letter). *J. Neurol. Neurosurg. Psychiatry*, **54** (9), 845–846.

Posner J, Cohen AF, Land G, Winton C and Peck AW (1989) The pharmacokinetics of lamotrigine (BW430C) in healthy subjects with unconjugated hyperbilirubinaemia (Gilbert's syndrome). *Br. J. Clin. Pharmacol.*, **28** (1), 117–120.

Ramsay RE, Pellock JM, Garnett WR et al. (1991) Pharmacokinetics and safety of lamotrigine (Lamictal) in patients with epilepsy. *Epilepsy Res.*, **10** (2–3), 191–200.

Richens A and Yuen AW (1991) Overview of the clinical efficacy of lamotrigine. *Epilepsia*, **32** (suppl. 2), S13–16.

Risner ME and the LAMICTAL Study Group (1990) Multicenter, double-blind, placebo controlled, add-on, crossover study of lamotrigene (Lamictal) in epileptic outpatients with partial seizures. *Epilepsia*, **31**, 619–620.

Rogawski MA and Porter RJ (1990) Antiepileptic drugs: pharmacological mechanisms and clinical efficacy with consideration of promising developmental stage compounds. *Pharmacol. Rev.*, **42**, 223–285.

Sailstad JM and Findlay JW (1991) Immunofluorometric assay for lamotrigine (Lamictal) in human plasma. *Ther. Drug Monit.*, **13** (5), 433–442.

Sander JW and Patsalos PN (1992) An assessment of serum and red blood cell folate concentrations in patients with epilepsy on lamotrigine therapy. *Epilepsy Res.*, **13** (1), 89–92.

Sander JW, Patsalos PN, Oxley JR, Hamilton MJ and Yuen WC (1990a) A randomised double-blind placebo-controlled add-on trial of lamotrigine in patients with severe epilepsy. *Epilepsy Res.*, **6** (3), 221–226.

Sander JW, Trevisol-Bittencourt PC, Hart YM, Patsalos PN and Shorvon SD (1990b) The efficacy and long-term tolerability of lamotrigine in the treatment of severe epilepsy. *Epilepsy Res.*, **7** (3), 226–229.

Schapel GJ, Beran RG, Vajda FJ et al. (1993) Double-blind, placebo controlled, crossover study of lamotrigine in treatment resistant partial seizures. *J. Neurol. Neurosurg. Psychiatry*, **56** (5), 448–453.

Schlumberger E, Chavez F, Palacios L, Rey E, Pajot N and Dulac O (1994) Lamotrigine in treatment of 120 children with epilepsy. *Epilepsia*, **35**, 359–367.

Sinz MW and Remmel RP (1991) Analysis of lamotrigine and lamotrigine 2-N-glucuronide in guinea pig blood and urine by reversed-phase ion-pairing liquid chromatography. *J. Chromatogr.*, **571** (1–2), 217–230.

Smith SE, al-Zubaidy ZA, Chapman AG and Meldrum BS (1993a) Excitatory amino acid antagonists, lamotrigine and BW 1003C87 as anticonvulsants in the genetically epilepsy-prone rat. *Epilepsy Res.*, **15** (2), 101–111.

Smith D, Baker G, Davies G, Dewey M and Chadwick DW (1993b) Outcomes of add-on treatment with lamotrigine in partial epilepsy. *Epilepsia*, **34** (2), 312–322.

Timmings PL and Richens A (1992) Lamotrigine as an add-on drug in the management of Lennox–Gastaut syndrome. *Eur. Neurol.*, **32** (6), 305–307.

Trnavska Z, Krejcova H, Tkaczykovam, Salcmanova Z and Elis J (1991) Pharmacokinetics of lamotrigine (Lamictal) in plasma and saliva. *Eur. J. Drug Metab. Pharmacokinet.*, Spec No. 3, 211–215.

Van Wieringen A, Binnie CD, De Boer PT, Van Emde Boas W, Overweg J and De Vries J (1987) Electroencephalographic findings in antiepileptic drug trials: a review and report of 6 studies. *Epilepsy Res.*, **1** (1), 3–15.

Van Wieringen A, Binnie CD, Meijer JW, Peck AW and de Vries J (1989) Comparison of the effects of lamotrigine and phenytoin on the EEG power spectrum and cortical and brainstem-evoked responses of normal human volunteers. *Neuropsychobiology*, **21**, 157–169.

Warner T, Patsalos PN, Prevett M, Elyas AA and Duncan JS (1992) Lamotrigine-induced carbamazepine toxicity: an interaction with carbamazepine-10,11-epoxide, *Epilepsy Res.*, **11** (2), 147–150.

Yuen AW (1991) Lamotrigine. *Epilepsy Res.*, **3** (suppl.), 115–123.

Yuen AW, Land G, Weatherley BC and Peck AW (1992) Sodium valproate acutely inhibits lamotrigine metabolism. *Br. J. Clin. Pharmacol.*, **33** (5), 511–513.

Zipp F, Baas H and Fischer PA (1993) Lamotrigine — antiparkinsonian activity by blockade of glutamate release? *J. Neural Transm. Park. Dis. Dement. Sect.*, **5** (1), 67–75.

# 7

# Oxcarbazepine

ANNE SABERS AND LENNART GRAM
*University Clinic of Neurology, Hvidovre Hospital, Denmark*

## INTRODUCTION

Carbamazepine is still one of the most important drugs for the treatment of patients with epilepsy. However, despite the excellent anticonvulsant effect of this drug, carbamazepine still has a number of disadvantages, such as acute dose-related toxicity, problems with development of rash and significant enzyme-inducing potential, causing problems in relation to concomitant treatment as well as a number of disturbing interactions. Consequently, improvement of this drug has been sought.

Oxcarbazepine was developed by manipulation of the chemical formula of carbamazepine with the aim of improving the tolerability profile without affecting the anticonvulsant potency.

About ten years of experience with oxcarbazepine in the treatment of epilepsy has placed this compound as a drug of first choice. The experience is based on more than 1300 patients participating in controlled studies as well as in open clinical trials.

Oxcarbazepine is marketed in several countries under the trade name Trileptal. The drug has already been the topic of several reviews and editorials (Gram and Philbert, 1986; Dam and Jensen, 1989; Editorial, 1989; Grant and Faulds, 1992).

This chapter deals only with the anticonvulsive aspects of oxcarbazepine, although the drug has clinical efficacy in the treatment of trigeminal neuralgia (Zakrzewska and Patsalos, 1989) as well as affective disorders (Emrich, 1990).

## PHARMACOLOGY

Oxcarbazepine, 10,11-dihydro-10-oxocarbamazepine, is the keto analogue of carbamazepine, chemically similar but with different metabolic pathways

*New Anticonvulsants: Advances in the Treatment of Epilepsy.* Edited by M. R. Trimble
© 1994 John Wiley & Sons Ltd

(Figure 1). It is rapidly and almost completely metabolized to the mono-hydroxy derivate (MHD) (10,11-dihydro-10-hydroxycarbamazepine) but without formation of the epoxide, which is considered to be responsible for some of the neurotoxic side-effects of carbamazepine. A minor amount of MHD is further transformed to the pharmacologically inactive dihydroxy derivative.

After ingestion, oxcarbazepine is almost completely absorbed from the gastrointestinal tract (Schütz *et al.*, 1986). As oxcarbazepine is rapidly and almost completely converted to the metabolite MHD, the pharmacokinetic aspects are primarily based on this active metabolite. MHD, as a lipophilic substance, is widely distributed in the body and easily passes the blood–brain barrier. The volume of distribution of MHD is about 0.3–0.8 l/kg (Feldmann *et al.*, 1981; Theisohn and Heimann, 1982). About 38% of MHD is bound to plasma proteins (Kristensen *et al.*, 1983).

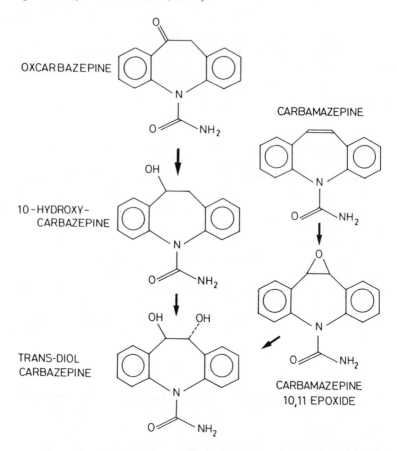

**Figure 1.**   Metabolism of carbamazepine and oxcarbazepine

The plasma elimination half-life of MHD lies in the range of 8–10 hours (Theisohn and Heimann, 1982) and appears stable on continued use of the drug, even in patients receiving concomitant anticonvulsants (Dickinson et al., 1989). More than 96% of oxcarbazepine is excreted by the kidneys, but less than 1% as unchanged drug (Schütz et al., 1986). There seems to be a considerable placental transfer of oxcarbazepine, as with most other anticonvulsant drugs. In a case reported by Bülau et al. (1988), maternal and neonatal plasma concentrations of oxcarbazepine were in the same range at delivery. The concentration ratio in breast milk and plasma was found to be about 0.5.

## DOSAGE AND PRACTICAL USE

Oxcarbazepine is only available for oral use. The less pronounced dose-related toxicity of oxcarbazepine means that dosage can be titrated much faster than carbamazepine to achieve the desired therapeutic response, one of the many advantages of this drug over carbamazepine.

The commonly recommended starting dose of oxcarbazepine in children is 10 mg/kg, with a stepwise increase to about 30 mg/kg. Adults may start with 600 mg per day and increase to a final daily dose in the range of 900–3000 mg. Elderly patients and patients with renal impairment probably require lower doses owing to a risk of decreased elimination rates of the drug (van Heiningen et al., 1991). As a result of the minor oxidative metabolism of oxcarbazepine the kinetics are not expected to be affected by impaired liver function. The glucuronide conjugate will, however, accumulate in patients with impaired kidney function.

In monotherapy, treatment with carbamazepine can be abruptly replaced by oxcarbazepine and vice versa; 300 mg of oxcarbazepine corresponds to 200 mg carbamazepine. However, in polytherapy, if oxcarbazepine is substituted for carbamazepine, there will be a loss of enzyme induction, and an acute rise of concomitant drugs. This may lead to toxicity. In such a setting, the changeover needs to be gradual, with appropriate serum level monitoring.

According to the half-life of the active metabolite, oxcarbazepine can be administered twice or three times a day. Tablets and syrup formulations can be exchanged without any need to adapt the existing dose regimen (Arnoldussen and Hulsman, 1988).

## THERAPEUTIC DRUG MONITORING

A definite therapeutic serum level for oxcarbazepine has not yet been established. On the basis of current evidence, a level of 50–125 µmol/l for the active metabolite has been suggested. Saliva drug levels have been suggested to be a useful method for monitoring oxcarbazepine (Kristensen *et al.*, 1983).

## DRUG INTERACTIONS

Problems with drug interactions often complicate concomitant treatment with more than one anticonvulsant drug. Many anticonvulsant drugs, including carbamazepine, induce liver microsomal cytochrome P450 oxygenases, resulting in enhanced metabolism of other drugs as well as autoinduction of their own metabolism. Elimination of oxcarbazepine and the active metabolite MHD are mainly catalysed by non-inducible cytosolic reductases (Faigle and Menge, 1990) and induction of the cytochrome P450 system in general is much less pronounced compared with carbamazepine. The reduced enzyme induction of oxcarbazepine makes polytherapy much simpler, since therapeutic blood levels of concomitant anticonvulsant drugs are easily obtained. Oxcarbazepine seems to decrease the bioavailability of the oestrogenic compounds of oral contraceptives, probably by induction of the P450 subgroup P450IIIA enzymes responsible for the metabolism of oestrogens. The study by Jensen *et al.* (1992) demonstrated breakthrough bleeding in 15% of healthy volunteers on a daily dose of 900 mg oxcarbazepine combined with oral contraceptives. Sonnen (1990) reported breakthrough bleeding in four of six women; this is comparable to the effect of carbamazepine.

The pharmacokinetics of oxcarbazepine and the active metabolite are not affected by erythromycin (Keränen *et al.*, 1992), by dextropropoxyphene (Mogensen *et al.*, 1992) or by cimetidine (Keränen *et al.*, 1990). In addition, the metabolism of warfarin is not influenced by oxcarbazepine (Krämer *et al.*, 1992).

## CLINICAL EFFICACY

### Controlled studies

The efficacy of oxcarbazepine has been evaluated in four randomized, double-blind studies in which the therapeutic potency of oxcarbazepine was compared mainly to the effect of carbamazepine. It should be noted that the severity of the epilepsies were different in these studies.

Houtkooper *et al.* (1987) compared the efficacy of oxcarbazepine and carbamazepine in a randomized, cross-over study with 48 hospitalized patients with various seizure types unsatisfactorily controlled on polytherapy. Concomitant treatments with phenytoin, valproate, ethosuximide, phenobarbitone or benzodiazepines were kept at constant doses during the trial.

During the oxcarbazepine treatment period a significant reduction of tonic–clonic seizures was observed.

The assessment of this result should be made with caution, since the shift from carbamazepine to oxcarbazepine was associated with a significant increase in the serum concentration of concomitant drugs, which was due to changes in hepatic enzyme induction during the trial. The mean daily dose of oxcarbazepine was 2628 mg (range 900–3600 mg), which was approximately double the carbamazepine dosage level of 1302 mg (range 500–2000 mg). The mean serum concentration of MHD was 98.3 μmol/l. No difference between the two drugs with regard to adverse effects was observed.

Bülau et al. (1987) undertook a comparative cross-over trial of carbamazepine and oxcarbazepine in 16 patients with epilepsy that was difficult to control despite treatment with carbamazepine and at least one additional anticonvulsant drug. The mean dose of carbamazepine was 1111 mg per day and that of carbazepine was 789 mg per day, with mean serum concentrations of carbamazepine 29 μmol/l and MHD 39 μmol/l. With regard to efficacy, no differences were observed in that approximately 25% of patients became seizure-free on both treatments. A non-significant trend towards fewer side-effects of oxcarbazepine was observed. However, the interpretation of this trial is difficult due to interactions, resulting in increased serum levels of concomitant drugs during oxcarbazepine treatment periods.

In 40 patients either refractory or intolerant to phenytoin, Reinikainen et al. (1987) randomly substituted either oxcarbazepine or carbamazepine for phenytoin. The mean duration of epilepsy in this group of patients was 12 years. An overall reduction of seizures was observed in both groups and there was no significant difference between the two treatment groups. However, with regard to side-effects a significant difference in favour of oxcarbazepine was established. This difference was especially observed during initiation of therapy. The nature of the adverse effects observed was similar for the two drugs. The dose of carbamazepine ranged from 400 mg to 800 mg per day, and that of oxcarbazepine from 600 mg to 900 mg per day. The serum concentrations of MDH were relatively low, 21–58 μmol/l, while carbamazepine levels were in the range 21–42 μmol/l.

In the Scandinavian multicentre trial (Dam et al., 1989), 235 drug-naive patients with newly diagnosed epilepsy were allocated to treatment with either oxcarbazepine or carbamazepine. The study comprised patients with partial seizures with or without secondary generalization. Of the patients treated with oxcarbazepine, 52% obtained complete seizure control, versus 60% in the carbamazepine group. The difference was not significant. In both groups more than 80% of the patients experienced at least 50% seizure reduction. However, with regard to toxicity a significant difference in favour of oxcarbazepine was demonstrated, since 'severe' adverse effects occurred significantly more frequently during treatment with carbamazepine. 'Severe' adverse effects were those that required treatment to be discontinued. Consequently, the global evaluation of tolerability by the investigators at the end of the study showed a non-significant trend in favour of oxcarbazepine. The mean dose of carbamazepine was 684 mg per day and for oxcarbazepine 1040 mg per day. The mean serum concentration of carbamazepine was 29.6 µmol/l and that of MHD was 57.0 µmol/l.

### Open studies

Nine years of experience with the use of oxcarbazepine were summarized in a large Danish retrospective multicentre study by Friis *et al.* (1993). In this study, 947 patients with various seizure types received oxcarbazepine to replace previous treatment (82%), as an adjunct to previous treatment (11%) or as the drug of first choice (7%); 63% of all patients received it as monotherapy. Compared with the three months before oxcarbazepine treatment, 51–66% experienced unchanged seizure frequency, 32–48% showed a decrease while 1–10% increased their seizure frequency. During treatment, 33% of all patients experienced side-effects, 18% necessitating withdrawal. Of the 350 patients whose electrolyte levels were monitored, 23% developed hyponatraemia. The study included all patients on oxcarbazepine treatment in eight participating centres, and included 67 patients aged less than 15 years. The mean maintenance was 30 mg/kg (range 7–87 mg/kg) in children and 18 mg/kg (range 4–61 mg/kg) in adults. Mean concentrations of MHD were 88 µmol/l in children, 79 µmol/l in adults and 68 µmol/l in elderly patients.

### TOLERABILITY

The development of oxcarbazepine by manipulation of the chemical formula of carbamazepine aimed at improving tolerability. Most studies therefore have focused on a comparison between the two drugs. Some adverse effects of carbamazepine seem to be associated with the active epoxide metabolite (Patsalos *et al.*, 1985; Rosenfield *et al.*, 1987). As oxcarbazepine undergoes metabolic reduction to the active MHD without epoxide formation, this lack of epoxidation therefore could explain the superior tolerability of oxcarbazepine compared with carbamazepine.

### Neurotoxicity

The most commonly reported side-effects are tiredness, headache, dizziness and ataxia (Houtkooper *et al.*, 1987; Reinikainen *et al.*, 1987; Dam *et al.*, 1989). The nature of side-effects is very similar during oxcarbazepine and carbamazepine treatment, but the number of side-effects seems to be greater in carbamazepine treatment. Dizziness seems to be more frequently reported during carbamazepine treatment compared with oxcarbazepine (Reinikainen et al., 1987).

Neuropsychological assessments revealed no measurable impairment of cognitive functions following four months and one year of oxcarbazepine monotherapy, respectively (Äikiä et al., 1992; Sabers et al., 1993).

**Systemic toxicity**

Except for a significant influence on serum sodium levels, oxcarbazepine-induced systemic side-effects are rare and transient. The drug may cause a mild increase of some liver enzymes (Bülau et al., 1987; Reinikainen et al., 1987; Friis et al., 1993), but the changes have no clinical significance and in no case lead to discontinuation of the drug.

Oxcarbazepine treatment, however, is frequently associated with the occurrence of hyponatraemia (Pendlebury et al., 1989). This effect is, as for carbamazepine, probably caused by an alteration in the normal regulation of antidiuretic hormone. However, the tendency seems to be more pronounced during oxcarbazepine treatment. In 41 patients on oxcarbazepine treatment, 21 exhibited serum sodium levels below 135 mmol/l (Nielsen et al., 1988). The hyponatraemic effect is usually mild and reversible, but increases at dosages higher than 25–30 mg/kg per day (Nielsen et al., 1988; Zakrzewska and Ivanyi, 1988). Hyponatraemia as a cause for discontinuation of oxcarbazepine is only occasionally reported (Friis et al., 1993). A case of water intoxication due to oxcarbazepine treatment showed complete reversibility upon discontinuation of the drug (Johannessen and Nielsen, 1987).

The electrocardiogram is not affected during oxcarbazepine treatment (Houtkooper et al., 1987).

**Idiosyncratic effects**

Allergic skin rashes seem to be less frequent during treatment with oxcarbazepine compared with carbamazepine (Houtkooper et al., 1987; Dam et al., 1989). In the prospective Scandinavian multicentre study (Dam et al., 1989), allergic side-effects led to withdrawal of the drug in 10% of the patients treated with oxcarbazepine compared with 16% in the carbamazepine group.

A study of cross-allergy between the two drugs has been undertaken (Jensen, 1985). The investigation comprised 51 patients with an allergic rash caused by carbamazepine. After switching to oxcarbazepine only 14 patients (27%) again developed an allergic rash. The vast majority (76%) of cases of rash occurred within the first month of treatment. It has been claimed that in vitro lymphocyte screening of cross-sensitivity of oxcarbazepine and carbamazepine may be useful (Zakrzewska and Ivanyi, 1988).

## OXCARBAZEPINE IN PREGNANCY

Experience with oxcarbazepine is still too limited to assess its teratogenic potential. However, it is reassuring that the drug has shown no teratogenic potential in animal studies, even at very high doses.

Of 12 women who received oxcarbazepine either as monotherapy or polytherapy, three had spontaneous abortion and nine had normal live-born children without congenital malformations (Friis et al., 1993). The rate of spontaneous abortion was not significantly higher than reports from the background population.

A case report by Bülau et al. (1988) described a mild facial dysmorphism with a discrete epicanthus and a somewhat broad-bridged nose, but no typical signs of an embryopathy. The child was developing normally when reexamined at the age of 13 months.


## CONCLUSION

Oxcarbazepine is a potent anticonvulsant drug comparable with other first-line anticonvulsant drugs with regard to efficacy. It is in general well tolerated, and severe adverse effects are relatively rare.

Oxcarbazepine was developed as a follow-up drug for carbamazepine. It has turned out to be as effective as carbamazepine and demonstrates a superior tolerability for the same therapeutic indications.

An additional advantage of oxcarbazepine is its minimal hepatic enzyme-inducing properties compared with many other anticonvulsant drugs, including carbamazepine. Except with regard to oral contraceptives, problems in relation to enzyme induction seem to have been eliminated. In addition, oxcarbazepine causes fewer interactions with other drugs compared with carbamazepine.

Instituting treatment with oxcarbazepine is much quicker and easier than with carbamazepine, because of its less pronounced dose-related toxicity.

Three out of four patients experiencing an allergic rash on carbamazepine will tolerate oxcarbazepine without developing cross-allergy.

A significant number of patients will develop hyponatraemia during oxcarbazepine treatment. However, almost all cases are non-symptomatic and fully reversible after reduction or discontinuation of the drug. Only occasionally will a patient have to discontinue treatment with this drug owing to symptoms caused by hyponatraemia.

Special attention should be paid to replacing carbamazepine with oxcarbazepine during anticonvulsant polytherapy, because this may cause an increase in the serum levels of concomitant drugs owing to different levels of enzyme induction.

# REFERENCES

Äikiä M, Kälviäinen R, Sivenius J, Halonen T and Riekkinen PJ (1992) Cognitive effects of oxcarbazepine and phenytoin monotherapy in newly diagnosed epilepsy: one year follow-up. *Epilepsy Res.*, **11**, 199–203.

Arnoldussen W and Hulsman J (1988) Oxcarbazepine (OCB) — a comparison of tablets versus syrup in epileptic children (abstract). *British, Danish and Dutch Epilepsy Congress*, Heemstede, 1988.

Bülau P, Stoll KD and Fröscher W (1987) Oxcarbazepine versus carbamazepine. In: *Advances in Epileptology* (eds P Wolf, M Dam, D Janz and FE Dreifuss), pp. 531–535. Raven Press, New York.

Bülau P, Paar WD and von Unruh GE (1988) Pharmacokinetics of oxcarbazepine and 10-hydroxy-carbazepine in the newborn child of an oxcarbazepine-treated mother. *Eur. J. Clin. Pharmac.*, **34**, 311–313.

Dam M and Jensen PK (1989) Oxcarbazepine. In: *Antiepileptic Drugs*, 3rd edn (eds RH Levy, FE Dreifuss, RH Mattson, BS Meldrum and JK Penry), pp. 913–924. Raven Press, New York.

Dam M, Ekberg R, Løyning Y, Waltimo O and Jacobsen K (1989) A double-blind study comparing oxcarbazepine and carbamazepine in patients with newly diagnosed, previously untreated epilepsy. *Epilepsy Res.*, **3**, 70–6.

Dickinson RG, Hooper WD, Dunstan PR and Eadie MJ (1984) First dose and steady-state pharmacokinetics of oxcarbazepine and its 10-hydroxy metabolite. *Eur. J. Clin. Pharmac.*, **37**, 69–74.

Editorial (1989) Oxcarbazepine. *Lancet,* **ii**, 196–198.

Emrich HM (1990) Studies with oxcarbazepine (Trileptal) in acute mania. *Int. Clin. Psychopharmacol.*, **5** (suppl. 1), 83–88.

Faigle JW and Menge GP (1990) Metabolic characteristics of oxcarbazepine (Trileptal) and their beneficial implications for enzyme induction and drug interactions. *Behav. Neurol.*, **3** (suppl. 1), 21–30.

Feldmann KF, Brechbühler S, Faigle JW and Imhof P (1981) Pharmacokinetics and metabolism of GP47779, the main human metabolite of oxcarbazepine (GP47680) in animals and healthy volunteers. In: *Advances in Epileptology: XIIth Epilepsy International Symposium* (eds M Dam, L Gram and JK Penry), pp. 89–96. Raven Press, New York.

Friis ML, Kristensen O, Boas J et al. (1993) Therapeutic experiences with 947 epileptic outpatients in oxcarbazepine treatment. *Acta Neurol. Scand.*, **87**, 224–227.

Gram L and Philbert A (1986) Oxcarbazepine. In: *New Anticonvulsant Drugs* (eds BS Meldrum and RJ Porter), pp. 229–235. John Libbey, London.

Grant SM and Faulds D (1992) Oxcarbazepine. A review of its pharmacology and therapeutic potential in epilepsy, trigeminal neuralgia and affective disorders. *Drugs*, **43**, 873–888.

Houtkooper MA, Lammertsma A, Meyer JWA et al. (1987) Oxcarbazepine (GP 47.680): a possible alternative to carbamazepine. *Epilepsia*, **28** (6), 693–698.

Jensen NO (1985) Oxcarbazepine in patients hypersensitive to carbamazepine. Paper presented at the 16th Epilepsy International Congress, Hamburg, 1985.

Jensen PK, Saano V, Haring P, Svenstrup B and Menge GP (1992) Possible interaction between oxcarbazepine and an oral contraceptive. *Epilepsia*, **33** (6), 1149–1152.

Johannessen AC and Nielsen OA (1987) Hyponatremia induced by oxcarbazepine. *Epilepsy Res.*, **1**, 155–156.

Keränen T, Jolkkonen J and Jensen PK (1990) Single-dose kinetics of oxcarbazepine after treatment with cimetidine or erythromycin. *Epilepsia*, **31**, 641.

Keränen T, Jolkkonen J, Jensen PK, Menge GP and Andersson P (1992) Absence of interactions between oxcarbazepine and erythromycin. *Acta Neurol. Scand.,* **86**, 120–131.

Krämer G, Tettenborn B, Jensen PK, Menga GP and Stoll KD (1992) Oxcarbazepine does not affect the anticoagulant activity of warfarin. *Epilepsia,* **33**, 1145–1148.

Kristensen O, Klitgaard NA, Jönsson B and Sindrup S (1983) Pharmacokinetics of 10-OH-carbazepine, the main metabolite of the antiepileptic oxcarbazepine, from serum and saliva concentrations. *Acta Neurol. Scand.,* **68**, 145–150.

Mogensen PH, Jørgensen L, Boas J et al. (1992) Effects of dextropropoxyphene on the steady-state kinetics of oxcarbazepine and its metabolites. *Acta Neurol. Scand.,* **85**, 14–17.

Nielsen OA, Johannessen AC and Bardrum B (1988) Oxcarbazepine-induced hyponatremia, a cross-sectional study. *Epilepsy Res.,* **2**, 269–271.

Patsalos PN, Stephenson TJ, Krishna S et al. (1985) Side-effects induced by carbamazepine 10,11 epoxide. *Lancet,* **i**, 496.

Pendlebury SC, Moses DK and Eadie MJ (1989) Hyponatremia during oxcarbazepine therapy. *Hum. Toxicol.,* **8**, 337–344.

Reinikainen KJ, Keränen T, Halonen T, Komulainen H and Riekkinen PJ (1987) Comparison of oxcarbazepine and carbamazepine: a double-blind study. *Epilepsy Res.,* **1**, 284–289.

Rosenfield WE, Holmes GB, Graves NM and Peterson AL (1987) Carbamazepine 10,11 epoxide serum concentration as a predictor of toxicity. *Epilepsia,* **28**, 580–581.

Sabers A and the Hvidovre Epilepsy Study Group (1993) Effect of monotherapeutic antiepileptic drugs on cognitive functions in patients with epilepsy (abstract). *Epilepsia,* **34** (suppl. 2), 11.

Schütz H, Feldmann KF, Faigle JW, Kriemler HP and Winkler T (1986) The metabolism of 14C-oxcarbazepine in man. *Xenobiotica,* **16** (8), 769–778.

Sonnen AEH (1990) Oxcarbazepine and oral contraceptives. *Acta Neurol. Scand.,* **82** (suppl. 133), 37.

Theisohn M and Heimann G (1982) Disposition of the antiepileptic oxcarbazepine and its metabolites in healthy volunteers. *Eur. J. Clin. Pharmac.,* **22**, 545–551.

van Heiningen P, Eve MD, Oosterhuis B et al. (1991) The influence of age on the antiepileptic agent oxcarbazepine. *Clin. Pharmacol. Therap.,* **50**, 410–419.

Zakrzewska JM and Ivanyi L (1988) In vitro lymphocyte proliferation by carbamazepine, carbamazepine-10,11-epoxide, and oxcarbazepine in the diagnosis of drug reduced hypersensitivity. *J. Allergy Clin. Immunol.,* **82**, 110–115.

Zakrzewska JM and Patsalos PN (1989) Oxcarbazepine: a new drug in the management of intractable trigeminal neuralgia. *J. Neurol. Neurosurg. Psychiatry,* **52**, 472–476.

# 8

# Vigabatrin

JOHN S. DUNCAN
*National Hospital for Neurology and Neurosurgery, London, UK*

## INTRODUCTION

Since the identification of gamma-aminobutyric acid (GABA) as a major inhibitory neurotransmitter in the central nervous system, attention has focused on how abnormalities of GABA transmission may underlie a propensity to epileptic seizures and how enhancement of GABAergic transmission may be used to inhibit seizures. It has, however, been recognized that the systemic administration of a drug to complex networks of dynamically interacting inhibitory and excitatory neurons may have unexpected consequences (Gale, 1989). Further, the action of GABA is not consistent in all types of epileptic seizure. While elevation of GABA concentrations inhibits the development of partial and secondarily generalized seizures (Meldum, 1984), this manoeuvre will increase the occurrence of generalized absences (Vergnes *et al.*, 1984; Peeters *et al.*, 1989).

## BIOCHEMISTRY AND PHARMACOLOGY

Vigabatrin (gamma-vinyl GABA) is a structural analogue of GABA and was designed to be a specific enzyme-activated suicide inhibitor of GABA transaminase, the principal enzyme that metabolizes GABA in glia and neurons (Lippert *et al.*, 1977). The drug is a racemic mixture and only the S(+) enantiomer is biologically active.

Vigabatrin forms a covalent bond with GABA transaminase and activity is only restored by synthesis of new enzyme. Administration of single doses of 1500 mg/kg of vigabatrin to rodents resulted in a decrease of brain GABA transaminase activity that reached a plateau within four hours and remained

*New Anticonvulsants: Advances in the Treatment of Epilepsy.* Edited by M. R. Trimble
© 1994 John Wiley & Sons Ltd

depressed for five days, with a parallel six-fold increase in total brain GABA concentrations (Jung *et al.*, 1977). The action of vigabatrin is specific and does not affect other aminotransferases. The reduction of glutamic acid decarboxylase activity that is noted *in vivo* but not *in vitro* appears to be a consequence of negative feedback exerted by the increased brain concentrations of GABA.

Administration of vigabatrin also results in increases in β-alanine (which is also a substrate for GABA transaminase) and homocarnosine concentrations (Schechter, 1986). There have been suggestions that vigabatrin may also function as a GABA reuptake blocker, and this may explain the immediate response seen in some patients when the drug is discontinued (Jolkonen *et al.*, 1992). In humans, clinically used doses of vigabatrin result in an elevation of cerebrospinal fluid GABA concentrations by approximately 150% (Riekkinen *et al.*, 1989).

Magnetic resonance spectroscopy has also been used to demonstrate the elevated concentration of GABA in the brain in rats receiving vigabatrin *in vivo* (Preece *et al.*, 1994) and also in human subjects (Rothman *et al.*, 1993). In the latter, clinically used doses of vigabatrin were associated with an approximately 200% rise in brain GABA concentrations. The non-invasive measurement of GABA concentrations in localized areas of brain holds much promise for gaining a better understanding of the pathophysiology of partial seizures and the effects of treatment. It has been postulated that patients who have a high level of glutamate in the cerebrospinal fluid have an increased chance of a good response to vigabatrin (Kalviainen *et al.*, 1993). It is possible that in the future the non-invasive assessment of neurotransmitter concentrations in the brain by magnetic resonance spectroscopy will allow the prospective identification of patients who are likely to benefit from vigabatrin.

Vigabatrin shows anticonvulsant activity in several animal models of epilepsy, including those in which derangement of GABAergic transmission is not thought to be involved in the pathogenesis of the seizures. It has been noted that there is often a poor correlation between total brain GABA concentration and efficacy. The likely explanation for this is that the anticonvulsant action is mediated by specific neuronal networks and that there is more than one pool of GABA in the brain (Schechter, 1986).

## PHARMACOKINETICS

Absorption from the gastrointestinal tract is rapid and almost total, with peak plasma concentrations in two hours. It has been suggested, on the basis of reduced plasma concentration curve integrals, that the bioavailability of oral vigabatrin may be less in young children than in adults (Rey *et al.*, 1990). The plasma concentration of the biologically active S(+) enantiomer is about 50%

of the concentration of the R(−) enantiomer (Haegele *et al.*, 1988). Vigabatrin in plasma is nearly all free, there is no appreciable protein binding.

Vigabatrin is excreted by the renal route, 70% being eliminated unchanged, with a half-life of five to seven hours in patients with normal renal function. A steady state is attained after a stable dosing regimen for two days. The elimination half-life and time taken to achieve a steady state are longer if there is impairment of renal function. In elderly subjects the slower rate of elimination of vigabatrin directly relates to reduced creatinine clearance.

## CLINICAL STUDIES OF EFFICACY OF VIGABATRIN

Nine double-blind studies (Rimmer and Richens, 1984; Gram *et al.*, 1985; Loiseau *et al.*, 1986; Remy *et al.*, 1986; Tartara *et al.*, 1986; Tassinari *et al.*, 1987; Ring *et al.*, 1990; McKee *et al.*, 1993; Grunewald *et al.*, 1994) and four single-blind studies (Gram *et al.*, 1983; Schechter *et al.*, 1984; Browne *et al.*, 1987; Cocito *et al.*, 1989) on a total of 218 and 133 patients respectively have been reported. Evaluation periods ranged from four weeks to 20 weeks, and the dose of vigabatrin from 1 g to 4 g, with 3 g per day being the most common. Overall, these studies have shown that about 50% of patients with refractory partial seizures show more than a 50% reduction in seizure frequency, and up to 10% may have complete seizure control. In general, most efficacy has been noted against complex partial seizures. There is little data on efficacy against primary generalized tonic–clonic seizures; one review suggests that vigabatrin is less effective against this seizure type than against partial seizures, with a 50% seizure reduction in 39% of patients (Michelucci and Tassinari, 1989). In an unblinded study of 45 children with infantile spasms, more than 50% had a greater than 50% reduction of spasms and seven of eight children with tuberous sclerosis had their spasms completely suppressed (Chiron *et al.* 1990). In another open study of 15 patients with infantile spasms, four became and remained seizure free, and four had a transient improvement with vigabatrin monotherapy (Appleton and Montiel-Viesca 1993). As yet no controlled studies of vigabatrin in infantile spasms have been reported.

Vigabatrin does not have any consistent effects on the electroencephalographic (EEG) background rhythms or on interictal epileptiform activity (Hammond and Wilder, 1985a; Ben-Menachem and Treiman, 1989; Mervaala *et al.*, 1989).

Long-term follow-up investigations of drug efficacy are difficult to interpret, as patients who do not do well tend to leave the study and so results often appear overoptimistic. Studies in which patients have been followed up for more than a year have suggested that a good response is maintained in over 60% of patients (Cocito *et al.*, 1989; Tartara *et al.*, 1989; Grunewald *et al.*, 1994), but tolerance may appear to develop in some patients (Sivenius *et al.*,

1991). Reynolds *et al.* (1991) did not find evidence for any loss of efficacy over a one-year follow-up of patients who showed an initial good response. In conclusion, it appears that most patients who show a favourable response to vigabatrin continue to do so.

Studies in progress include a parallel comparison of vigabatrin monotherapy with carbamazepine in patients with newly diagnosed partial seizures (Kalviainen *et al.*, 1993) and a comparison with sodium valproate in patients whose partial seizures have not been adequately controlled with carbamazepine.

**Patients with mental retardation**

Thirteen of 30 patients with partial seizures and two of six patients with primary generalized epilepsy had a greater than 50% reduction of seizures in an open study of patients with mental handicap (Matilainen *et al.*, 1988). In 33% of patients who responded initially, the benefit was lost over a five-year follow-up (Pitkanen *et al.*, 1993).

## CURRENT INDICATIONS

Vigabatrin is a second-line drug for partial seizures and secondary generalized tonic–clonic seizures. Vigabatrin may also be useful against other seizure types, with the exception of generalized absences and myoclonus, which may be markedly exacerbated (Loscher, 1982). In general, a beneficial effect of vigabatrin is usually maintained but tolerance may develop in some patients who show an initial response.

Experience in idiopathic generalized epilepsy is limited; efficacy against generalized tonic–clonic seizures appears to be less than that against partial seizures, and there is anecdotal evidence of worsening of absences and myoclonic seizures that may be part of the idiopathic generalized epilepsy syndrome.

## MEASUREMENT OF PLASMA CONCENTRATIONS

The plasma concentration of vigabatrin appears to bear a linear relationship to the ingested dose, at least for single doses in the clinical range. However, as vigabatrin functions as an irreversible inhibitor of GABA transaminase the biological effect of the drug lasts for much longer than the drug is detectable in the plasma. In consequence, the plasma concentrations of vigabatrin do not relate well to clinical efficacy or the development of adverse effects. The initially proposed target range of plasma concentrations was 40–270 µmol/l. As a result, measurement of plasma concentrations of vigabatrin is not useful as a guide to dosing, but may be used as a check on recent compliance.

Vigabatrin has been shown to inhibit the activity of GABA transaminase in platelets (Bolton *et al.*, 1989). To date, this has not been shown to be a useful guide to drug dosage (Arteaga *et al.*, 1992).

In elderly patients and in those with renal impairment, the measurement of plasma concentrations may have a role in ensuring that very high levels of the drug are not developing.

## DOSING

A usual starting dose for an adult is 500 mg, once or twice a day, increasing in 500 mg steps every one to two weeks. Average maintenance doses are 1–1.5 g twice daily. About 25% of patients have better control on 3 g than on 2 g; conversely, some patients seem to be better controlled on the lower dose. In general, there appears to be no benefit from increasing doses beyond 3–4 g per day. In children, 40 mg/kg per day is a usual starting dose, with maintenance doses of 80–100 mg/kg per day. Lower doses should be used in patients with renal impairment, particularly when the creatinine clearance is less than 60 ml/min.

In clinical trials, the abrupt cessation of vigabatrin has been associated with a marked increase in seizures (Ring *et al.*, 1990; Sander *et al.*, 1990) and tapering of the drug over three to four weeks is recommended, unless there are grounds for attempting to discontinue the drug more quickly, such as the development of a severe adverse effect.

### Interval between doses

In view of the prolonged biological effect of vigabatrin, once or twice daily dosing appears satisfactory. Many patients prefer to take vigabatrin in two doses per day, because of the bulk of the medication. In some early studies the efficacy of alternate day dosing appeared to be less good than with daily administration; this was probably because of the reduced total dose administered with dosing on alternate days (Ben-Menachem *et al.*, 1989).

## DRUG INTERACTIONS

The virtual lack of pharmacokinetic interactions between vigabatrin and other anticonvulsant drugs is a distinct advantage for a drug that is almost invariably added to existing therapy.

### Effect of other drugs on vigabatrin

No other medications, whether anticonvulsant drugs or other therapeutic agents, appear to have a significant pharmacokinetic or pharmacodynamic effect on vigabatrin. There have been anecdotal reports of a synergistic action with lamotrigine, but there are no controlled data to substantiate this.

### Effect of vigabatrin on other drugs

In patients taking phenytoin, the addition of vigabatrin results in a fall in the plasma concentrations of phenytoin by an average of 20–30% (Rimmer and Richens, 1984; Browne et al., 1987; Tartara et al., 1989; Patsalos and Duncan, 1993). This effect is generally noted about one month after the addition of vigabatrin to phenytoin. This interaction does not involve phenytoin plasma protein binding or metabolism and the mechanism is not established. One postulate is that the bioavailability of phenytoin is reduced, but this is not certain. In the majority of patients this interaction is not of clinical significance, but occasionally a corrective increase in phenytoin dose may be necessary if there is an impairment of seizure control at this time. The corollary of this effect is that plasma phenytoin concentrations rise by an average of 20–30% after the withdrawal of vigabatrin therapy.

The plasma concentrations of phenobarbitone and primidone may also occasionally appear to be reduced a few weeks after the addition of vigabatrin to these medications. This is not a consistent finding, however, and in general does not appear to be of any clinical significance. There is usually no significant change in the plasma concentrations of carbamazepine or sodium valproate consequent to the addition or withdrawal of vigabatrin.

## ADVERSE EFFECTS

### Acute and idiosyncratic adverse effects

Sedation, dizziness and headache are the most commonly reported acute adverse effects, particularly when doses are being increased. Ataxia and tremor also occur. Tolerance often develops and the symptoms are frequently self-limiting. To a large extent these symptoms can be avoided by introducing the drug gradually, so that a dose of 3 g per day is reached after gradual increments over five weeks. Allergic skin rashes are extremely rare.

### Neuropsychiatric adverse effects

Up to one patient in 10 develops a change in mood, commonly agitation, ill-temper and disturbed behaviour, or depression. Overall, up to 4% of patients receiving vigabatrin may develop paranoid and psychotic symptoms (Sander and Hart, 1990; Sander et al., 1991), although other groups have found a lower incidence (Betts and Thomas, 1990; Dam, 1990). The onset of psychosis has generally occurred 1–36 weeks after starting treatment. The doses of vigabatrin taken by affected patients have not been particularly high. Some patients have become psychotic after developing a respite from seizures, and in others this has occurred after a cluster of seizures. There have also been reports of psychosis developing after abrupt discontinuation of vigabatrin (Brodie and McKee, 1990; Ring and Reynolds, 1990).

Depression has been noted to develop in 4–9% of patients receiving vigabatrin in double-blind studies (Rimmer and Richens, 1984; Gram et al., 1985; Loiseau et al., 1986; Remy et al., 1986; Tartara et al., 1986; Tassinari et al., 1987; Grunewald et al., 1994). Depression has generally been noted when the drug is being introduced or following a subsequent dose increase. A past history of psychiatric disturbance appears to increase the risk of developing depression (Ring et al., 1993) and such patients should be kept under close review.

The incidence of severe psychiatric and behavioural adverse effects appears to have reduced since the recognition of this problem in 1990, most probably because of the trend towards slower introduction of the drug and awareness of the initial symptoms of psychiatric disturbance, which resolve on dose reduction. In most patients in whom adverse psychiatric and behavioural effects occur, the symptoms evolve over several days and serious problems may generally be averted if drug usage is tapered off. In clinical practice it is clearly important to warn patients, carers and primary care physicians of the possible adverse effects, and to give advice on reducing the medication should these occur.

### Cognitive function

Effects on cognitive function have been assessed by several studies with the conclusion that there is no adverse effect (Mumford et al., 1990; McGuire et al., 1992; Gillham et al., 1993) or a slight slowing on a test of motor function and impairment on a measure of visual memory (Grunewald et al., 1994).

### Other chronic adverse effects

Weight gain of 10 kg or more occurs in about 15% of adults and may limit the acceptability of the drug, even if seizure control is significantly improved. Tartara et al. (1989) reported that 40% of their patients had a weight gain of 5–16% during the first three to six months of therapy, with a subsequent levelling off of weight gain.

### Teratogenicity

There is very little data on the teratogenic potential of vigabatrin. Animal studies were generally satisfactory, with the only abnormality being an increased incidence of cleft palate in rabbits. To date there have been 22 reported live births to women who have taken vigabatrin throughout pregnancy. There is no evidence so far of any marked teratogenic effect, but with such small numbers, conclusions are only very tentative.

### Neuropathological studies

Neuropathological studies in rats and dogs raised a concern about the development of intramyelinic oedema and reactive astrocytosis that was related to administration of vigabatrin (Butler et al., 1987; Gibson et al., 1990). Monkeys who were administered a maximal tolerated dose of 300 mg/kg per day for 16 months produced equivocal changes only (Gibson et al., 1990). In dogs and rats this pathology is detectable non-invasively in vivo, with magnetic resonance imaging (MRI) showing prolongation of T2 relaxation time and increased T2-weighted signal intensity (Jackson et al., 1991; Sussman et al., 1991). It has also been shown that quantitation of T2 relaxation times is more sensitive and reproducible than qualitative inspection of MR images (Jackson et al., 1991). In dogs, the development of intramyelinic oedema was paralleled by prolongation of visual and somatosensory evoked response latencies (Arezzo et al., 1989; Schroeder et al., 1992).

Data from patients treated with vigabatrin have been reassuring. Evoked responses in treated patients have not been prolonged (Hammond and Wilder, 1985b; Cosi et al., 1989; Liegois-Chauvel et al., 1989; Mervaala et al., 1989; Ylinen et al., 1992). A prospective double-blind evaluation of the effects of 3 g per day of vigabatrin for four months, and subsequent open follow-up for up to 18 months, did not find any prolongation of T2 relaxation times using quantitative MRI, which might have been suggestive of the development of intramyelinic oedema and astrocytosis, over these periods (Grunewald et al., 1993). Less rigorous qualitative MRI studies have also not shown any changes suggestive of intramyelinic oedema (Chiron et al., 1989; Cocito et al., 1992).

Further, postmortem examination of the brains of more than 11 patients who died while taking vigabatrin, and findings in over 50 surgical excision specimens (Pedersen et al., 1987; Ben-Menachem et al., 1988; Trottier et al., 1989; Agosti et al., 1990; Paljarvi et al., 1990; Cannon et al., 1991; Hammond et al., 1992; Sivenius et al., 1993) have not suggested that this phenomenon occurs with clinically used doses in patients. In spite of the reassuring data so far obtained, vigilance needs to be maintained to assess the possible development of neuropathological changes over longer treatment periods. One remaining caveat is that in rats, reactive astrocytosis *without* concomitant intramyelinic oedema was noted in cerebral cortex and thalamus (Jackson et al., 1991), and the significance of this feature may be difficult to evaluate in patients with epilepsy and pre-existing cerebral damage and gliosis.

## CONCLUSION

Of all the anticonvulsant drugs introduced in the last five years, vigabatrin has the most efficacy against partial seizures that have proved refractory to treatment with more established agents. This potency carries with it a potential for psychiatric adverse effects. However, awareness of this possible problem, the use of gradual dose escalation and decrease, and appropriate anticipatory action in the event of any adverse change of mood or behaviour appear to have reduced the risk of serious adverse effects.

The current place of vigabatrin is as a second-line drug for patients with refractory partial and secondary generalized tonic–clonic seizures. Vigabatrin may also be useful against other seizure types, with the exception of absences and myoclonus, which may be markedly exacerbated. This last fact greatly limits the utility of vigabatrin in patients with idiopathic generalized epilepsy. Preliminary studies suggest that vigabatrin may be very beneficial against infantile spasms.

In general a beneficial effect of vigabatrin is usually maintained, but tolerance may develop in some patients who show an initial response. Vigabatrin is an easy drug to prescribe and to take. There is little risk of a significant pharmacokinetic interaction with other drugs and there is no need to measure the plasma concentration as a guide to dosing, although this investigation may be helpful in patients with renal impairment.

## REFERENCES

Agosti R, Yasurgil G, Egli M, Wieser HG and Wiestler OD (1990) Neuropathology of a human hippocampus following long-term treatment with vigabatrin: lack of microvacuoles. *Epilepsy Res.*, **6**, 166–170.

Appleton RE, Montiel-Viesca F (1993) Vigabatrin in infantile spasms — why add on? *Lancet*, **341**, 962.

Arezzo JC, Schroeder CE, Litwak MS and Steward DL (1989) Effects of vigabatrin on evoked potentials in dogs. *Br. J. Clin. Pharmacol.*, **27** (suppl. 1), 53S–60S.

Arteaga R, Herranz JL, Valdizan EM and Armijo JA (1992) Gamma-vinyl GABA (vigabatrin): relationship between dosage, plasma concentrations, platelet GABA-transaminase inhibition, and seizure reduction in epileptic children. *Epilepsia*, **33**, 923–931.

Ben-Menachem E and Treiman DM (1989) Effect of gamma-vinyl GABA on interictal spikes and sharp waves in patients with intractable complex partial seizures. *Epilepsia*, **30**, 79–83.

Ben-Menachem E, Nordborg C, Hedstrom A, Augustinsson L-E and Silvenius H (1988) Case report of a surgical brain sample after 2½ years of vigabatrin therapy. *Epilepsia*, **29**, 699.

Ben-Menachem E, Persson LI, Schechter PJ *et al.* (1989) The effect of different vigabatrin treatment regimens on CSF biochemistry and seizure control in epileptic patients. *Br. J. Clin. Pharmacol.* **27** (suppl. 1), 79S–85S.

Betts T and Thomas L (1990) Vigabatrin and behaviour disturbances. *Lancet*, **335**, 1279.

Bolton JB, Rimmer E, Williams J and Richens A (1989) The effect of vigabatrin on brain and platelet GABA-transaminase activities. *Br. J. Clin. Pharmacol.*, **27**, 35S.

Brodie MJ and McKee PJW (1990) Vigabatrin and psychosis. *Lancet*, **335**, 1279.

Browne TR, Mattson RH, Penry JK *et al.* (1987) Vigabatrin for complex partial seizures: multicenter single-blind study with long-term follow-up. *Neurology*, **37**, 184–189.

Butler WH, Ford GP and Newberne JWA (1987) Study of the effects of vigabatrin on the central nervous system and retina of Sprague Dawley and Lister-hooded rats. *Toxicol. Pathol.*, **15**, 143–148.

Cannon DJ, Butler WH, Mumford JP and Lewis PJ (1991) Neuropathologic findings in patients receiving long-term vigabatrin therapy for chronic intractable epilepsy. *J. Child Neurol.*, **6** (suppl. 2), 2S17–2S24.

Chiron C, Dulac O, Palacios L *et al.* (1989) Magnetic resonance imaging in epileptic children treated with γ-vinyl GABA (vigabatrin). *Epilepsia*, **30** (suppl. 1), 736.

Chiron C, Dulac O, Luna D *et al.* (1990) Vigabatrin in infantile spasms. *Lancet*, **335**, 363–364.

Cocito L, Maffini M, Perfumo P *et al.* (1989) Vigabatrin in complex partial seizures: a long-term study. *Epilepsy Res.*, **3**, 160–166.

Cocito L, Maffini M and Loeb C (1992) MRI findings in epileptic patients on vigabatrin for more than 5 years. *Seizure*, **1**, 163–165.

Cosi V, Callieco R, Galimberti CA *et al.* (1989) Effects of vigabatrin on evoked potentials in epileptic patients. *Br. J. Clin. Pharmacol.*, **27**, 61S–68S.

Dam M (1990) Vigabatrin and behaviour disturbances. *Lancet*, **335**, 605.

Gale K (1989) GABA in epilepsy: the pharmacologic basis. *Epilepsia*, **30** (suppl. 3), S1–S11.

Gibson JP, Yarrington JT, Loudy DE, Gerbig CG, Hurst GH and Newberne JW (1990) Chronic toxicity studies with vigabatrin, a GABA-transaminase inhibitor. *Toxicol. Pathol.*, **18**, 225–238.

Gillham RA, Blacklaw J, McKee PJW and Brodie MJ (1993) Effect of vigabatrin on sedation and cognitive function in patients with refractory epilepsy. *J. Neurol. Neurosurg. Psychiatry*, **56**, 1271–1275.

Gram L, Blatt Lyon B and Dam M (1983) Gamma-vinyl GABA: a single blind trial in patients with epilepsy. *Acta Neurol. Scand.*, **68**, 34–39.

Gram L, Klosterkov P and Dam M (1985) Gamma-vinyl GABA: a double-blind placebo-controlled trial in partial epilepsy. *Ann. Neurol.*, **17**, 262–266.

Grunewald RA, Jackson GD, Connelly A and Duncan JS (1993) Vigabatrin-related changes in the human brain measured by quantitative MRI. *Epilepsia*, **34** (suppl. 6), 97.

Grunewald RA, Thompson PJ, Corcoran RS, Corden Z, Jackson GD and Duncan JS (1994) Effects of vigabatrin on partial seizures and cognitive function. *J. Neurol. Neurosurg. Psychiatry* (in press).

Haegele K, Huebert ND, Ebel M, Tell G and Schechter PJ (1988) Pharmacokinetics of vigabatrin: implications of creatinine clearance. *Clin. Pharmacol. Therap.*, **44**, 558.

Hammond EJ and Wilder BJ (1985a) Effects of gamma-vinyl GABA on the human electroencephalogram. *Neuropharmacology*, **24**, 975–984.

Hammond EJ and Wilder BJ (1985b) Effect of gamma-vinyl GABA on human pattern evoked visual potentials. *Neurology*, **35**, 1801–1803.

Hammond EJ, Ballinger WE, Lu L, Wilder BJ, Uthman BM and Reid SA (1992) Absence of cortical white matter changes in three patients undergoing long-term vigabatrin therapy. *Epilepsy Res.,* **12**, 261–265.

Jackson GD, Williams SR, van Bruggen N, Williams SCR and Duncan JS (1991) Vigabatrin-induced cerebellar and cortical lesions are demonstrated by quantitative MRI. *Epilepsia,* **32** (suppl. 1), 13.

Jolkonen J, Mazurkiewicz M, Lahtinen H and Riekkinen PJ (1992) Acute effects of gamma-vinyl GABA on the GABAergic system in rats as studied by microdialysis. *Eur. J. Pharmacol.,* **229**, 269–272.

Jung MJ, Lippert B, Metcalf BW, Bohlen P and Schechter PJ (1977) γ-vinyl GABA (4-amino-hex-5-enoic acid): a new selective irreversible inhibitor of GABA-T: effects on brain GABA metabolism in mice. *J. Neurochem.,* **29**, 797–802.

Kalviainen R, Halonen T, Pitkanen A and Riekkinen PJ (1993) Amino acid levels in the cerebrospinal fluid of newly diagnosed epileptic patients: effect of vigabatrin and carbamazepine monotherapies. *J. Neurochem.,* **60**, 1244–1250.

Liegois-Chauvel C, Marquis P, Gisselbrecht D *et al.* (1989) Effects of long-term vigabatrin on somatosensory-evoked potentials in epileptic patients. *Epilepsia,* **30** (suppl. 3), S23–S25.

Lippert B, Metcalf BW, Jung MJ and Casara P (1977) 4-amino-hex-5-enoic acid: a selective catalytic inhibitor of 4-aminobutyric-acid transferase in mammalian brain. *Eur. J. Biochem.,* **74**, 441–445.

Loiseau P, Hardenberg JP, Pestre M *et al.* (1986) Double-blind placebo-controlled study of vigabatrin (Gamma-vinyl GABA) in drug-resistant epilepsy. *Epilepsia,* **27**, 115–120.

Loscher W (1982) Comparative assay of anticonvulsant and toxic properties of sixteen GABAmimetic drugs. *Neuropharmacology,* **21**, 803–810.

Matilainen R, Pitkanen A, Ruutiaienen T *et al.* (1988) Effect of vigabatrin on epilepsy in mentally retarded patients: a 7 month follow-up study. *Neurology,* **38**, 743–747.

McGuire AM, Duncan JS and Trimble MR (1992) Effects of vigabatrin on cognitive function and mood, when used as add-on therapy in patients with intractable epilepsy. *Epilepsy,* **33**, 128–134.

McKee PJW, Blacklaw J, Friel E, Thompson GG, Gillham RA and Brodie MJ (1993) Adjuvant vigabatrin in refractory epilepsy: a ceiling to effective dosage in individual patients? *Epilepsia,* **34**, 937–943.

Meldum BS (1984) Amino acid neurotransmitters and new approaches to anticonvulsant drug action. *Epilepsia,* **25** (suppl. 2), S140–S149.

Mervaala E, Partanen J, Nousiainen U *et al.* (1989) Electrophysiological effects of gamma-vinyl GABA and carbamazepine. *Epilepsia,* **30**, 189–193.

Michelucci R and Tassinari CA (1989) Response to vigabatrin in relation to seizure type. *Br. J. Clin. Pharmacol.,* **27** (suppl. 1), 119S–124S.

Mumford JP, Beaumont D and Gisselbrecht D (1990) Cognitive function, mood and behaviour in vigabatrin treated patients. *Acta Neurol. Scand.,* **82** (suppl. 133), 15.

Paljarvi L, Vapalahti M, Sivenius J and Riekkinen P (1990) Neuropathological findings in five patients with vigabatrin treatment. *Neurology,* **40** (suppl. 1), 153.

Patsalos PN and Duncan JS (1993) Antiepileptic drugs: a review of clinically significant interactions. *Drug Safety,* **9**, 156–184.

Pedersen B, Hojgaard K and Dam M (1987) Vigabatrin: no microvacuoles in a human brain. *Epilepsy Res.,* **1**, 74–76.

Peeters BWMM, van Rijn CM, Vossen JHM and Coenen AML (1989) Effects of GABA-ergic agents on spontaneous non-convulsive epilepsy, EEG and behaviour in the WAG/Rij strain. *Life Sci.,* **45**, 1171–1176.

Pitkanen A, Ylinen A, Matilainen R *et al.* (1993) Long-term antiepileptic efficacy of vigabatrin in drug-refractory epilepsy in mentally retarded patients. A 5-year follow-up study. *Arch. Neurol.,* **50**, 24–29.

Preece NA, Jackson GD, Houseman JA, Duncan JS and Williams SR (1994) NMR detection of elevated cortical GABA in the vigabatrin-treated rat in vivo. *Epilepsia* (in press).

Remy C, Favel P, Tell G *et al.* (1986) Etude en double aveugle contre placebo en permutations croisées du vigabatrin dans l'épilepsie de l'adulte résistant à la thérapeutique. *Boll. Lega. It. Epil.,* **54/55**, 241–243.

Rey E, Pons G, Richard MO, Vauzelle F *et al.* (1990) Pharmacokinetics of the individual enantiomers of vigabatrin (gamma-vinyl-GABA) in epileptic children. *Br. J. Clin. Pharmacol.,* **30**, 253.

Reynolds EH, Ring HA, Farr IN, Heller AJ and Elwes RDC (1991) Open, double blind and long term study of vigabatrin in chronic epilepsy. *Epilepsia,* **32**, 530–538.

Riekkinen PJ, Ylinen A, Halonen T *et al.* (1989) Cerebrospinal fluid GABA and seizure control with vigabatrin. *Br. J. Clin. Pharmacol.,* **27** (suppl. 1), 87S–94S.

Rimmer EM and Richens A (1984) Double-blind study of gamma-vinyl GABA in patients with refractory epilepsy. *Lancet,* **ii**, 189–190.

Ring HA and Reynolds EH (1990) Vigabatrin and behaviour disturbance. *Lancet,* **335**, 970.

Ring HA, Heller AJ, Farr IN and Reynolds EH (1990) Vigabatrin: rational treatment for chronic epilepsy. *J Neurol. Neurosurg. Psychiatry,* **53**, 1051–1053.

Ring HA, Crellin R, Kirker S and Reynolds EH (1993) Vigabatrin and depression. *J. Neurol. Neurosurg. Psychiatry,* **56**, 925–928.

Rothman DL, Petroff OAC, Behar KL and Mattson RH (1993) Localized $^1$H NMR measurements of γ-aminobutyric acid in human brain *in vivo. Proc. Natl Acad. Sci. USA,* **90**, 5662–5666.

Sander JWAS and Hart YM (1990) Vigabatrin and behaviour disturbance. *Lancet,* **335**, 57.

Sander JWAS, Trevisol-Bittencourt PC, Hart YM and Shorvon SD (1990) Evaluation of vigabatrin as an add-on drug in the management of severe epilepsy. *J. Neurol. Neurosurg. Psychiatry,* **53**, 1008–1010.

Sander JWAS, Hart YM, Trimble MR and Shorvon SD (1991) Vigabatrin and psychosis. *J. Neurol. Neurosurg. Psychiatry,* **54**, 435–439.

Schechter PJ (1986) Vigabatrin. In: *Current Problems in Epilepsy: New Anticonvulsant Drugs* (eds BS Meldrum and RJ Porter), Vol. 4, pp. 265–275. John Libbey, London.

Schechter PJ, Hanke NF, Grove J *et al.* (1984) Biochemical and clinical effects of gamma-vinyl GABA in patients with epilepsy. *Neurology,* **34**, 182–186.

Schroeder CE, Gibson JP, Yarrington J, Heydorn WE, Sussman NM and Arezzo JC (1992) Effects of high dose γ-Vinyl-GABA (Vigabatrin) administration on visual and somatosensory evoked potentials in dogs. *Epilepsia,* **33** (suppl. 5), S13–S25.

Sivenius J, Ylinen A, Murros K, Mumford JP and Riekkinen PJ (1991) Vigabatrin in drug resistant partial epilepsy: a 5 year follow-up study. *Neurology,* **41**, 562–565.

Sivenius J, Paljarvi L, Vapalahti M and Riekkinen P (1993) Vigabatrin (γ-Vinyl-GABA): neuropathologic evaluation in five patients. *Epilepsia,* **34**, 193–196.

Sussman NM, Weiss KL, Schroeder CE *et al.* (1991) Vigabatrin: effects on in vivo and ex vivo magnetic resonance imaging of dog brains. *Epilepsia,* **32** (suppl. 1), 13.

Tartara A, Manni R, Galimberti CA *et al.* (1986) Vigabatrin in the treatment of epilepsy: a double-blind placebo-controlled study. *Epilepsy,* **27**, 717–723.

Tartara A, Manni R, Galimberti CA, Mumford JP, Iudice A and Perucca E (1989) Vigabatrin in the treatment of epilepsy: a long-term follow-up study. *J. Neurol. Neurosurg. Psychiatry,* **52**, 467–471.

Tassinari CA, Michelucci R, Ambrosetto G and Salvi F (1987) Double-blind study of vigabatrin in the treatment of drug-resistant epilepsy. *Arch. Neurol.,* **44**, 907–910.

Trottier S, Hauw JJ, Chauvel P, Chodkiewicz JP and Beaumont D (1989) Neuropathological examination of brain tissue in patients treated with vigabatrin. *Adv. Epileptol.,* **17**, 166–168.

Vergnes M, Marescaux C, Micheletti G, Depaulis A, Rumbach L and Warter JM (1984) Enhancement of spike and wave discharges by GABAmimetic drugs in rats with spontaneous petit mal-like epilepsy. *Neurosi. Lett.,* **44**, 91–94.

Ylinen A, Sivenius J, Pitkanen A *et al.* (1992) γ-vinyl GABA (vigabatrin) in epilepsy: clinical, neurochemical, and neurophysiologic monitoring in epileptic patients. *Epilepsia,* **35**, 917–922.

# 9

# The use of new anticonvulsant drugs in children

JOHN M. PELLOCK
*Medical College of Virginia, Richmond, Virginia, USA*

Although epilepsy in childhood is frequently well controlled by existing anti-convulsant drugs, more than 25% of paediatric patients have uncontrolled seizures, truly intractable seizures or significant adverse effects (Pellock, 1989; Dodson, 1993a; Heller *et al.*, 1993). Certain children with epilepsy who do not respond to medication should be considered for surgical treatment. However, this group is limited in number, and the quest for more efficacious medications that may have fewer adverse effects and allow a better quality of life must continue. Because certain seizure types are more common or only appear in childhood, specific medications are required to treat these special syndromes (Roger *et al.*, 1992; Pellock, 1993). On the other hand, partial seizures which are present in childhood seem to respond to medications used for the control of partial seizures in adults. There is no evidence that the mechanisms of partial epilepsy in children or the anticonvulsant drugs used to treat these partial seizures differ from those in adults. Figure 1 demonstrates the major age-related epilepsy syndromes of childhood.

The study of paediatric clinical pharmacology of anticonvulsant drugs has clearly demonstrated that children utilize drugs differently from adults (Dodson and Pellock, 1993). Each child's dosage should be individualized, because children vary widely in their ability to eliminate drugs, even more so than adults. In general, following the newborn period, children demonstrate rapid hepatic metabolism and good renal clearance. The therapy of child epilepsy is less predictable and more time-consuming than that of adults, and may involve trial and error. Understanding the pharmacokinetics of anticonvulsant drugs in children requires not only an immediate assessment of pharmacokinetics, but also consideration of what will happen as the child develops. Thus, when newer anticonvulsants are being considered for use in children, an evaluation of

*New Anticonvulsants: Advances in the Treatment of Epilepsy*. Edited by M. R. Trimble
© 1994 John Wiley & Sons Ltd

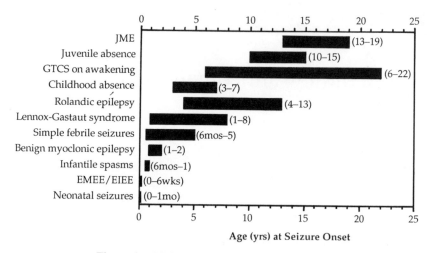

**Figure 1.**   Major age related epilepsy syndromes

special pharmacokinetic and safety issues must be undertaken. Both active and inactive metabolites should be considered and special safety and adverse effect profiles should be developed in children (Commission on Antiepileptic Drugs of the International League Against Epilepsy, 1991).

The following section demonstrates how, in general, the newer anticonvulsant drugs have been developed for use in adults initially, with only smaller studies being done for safety in children. Efficacy studies in special types of childhood epilepsy usually follow the establishing of safety and efficacy data in adults. No large-scale, controlled studies using older or newer anticonvulsants have been performed in neonatal seizures or most of the malignant childhood epilepsies (progressive myoclonic epilepsy, Kojewnikow's syndrome, etc.). A summary of childhood epilepsy studies involving the newer drugs (in alphabetical order) is given below.

## CLOBAZAM

There are a few open studies of the use of clobazam in children. Farrell (1986) has reviewed these in more detail. He noted the more extensive use of benzodiazepines generally in myoclonic and atonic seizures and as adjunctive therapy in the treatment of atypical absence seizures. He reported on the use of clobazam as adjunctive therapy in 50 children with refractory epilepsy, aged 2–16 years. The majority had mental retardation, and 33 had the Lennox–Gastaut syndrome. Clobazam was added to the existing regimen at a dose of 5 mg per day and increased at five-day intervals to a maximum of 40 mg per day. Thirty-four per cent of patients responded initially and then showed tolerance within four months of starting the drug. In the majority of these, there was only partial relapse. Seizures were controlled completely in 20%, and improved markedly in a further 34%. With regard to seizure type, atypical absence seizures were controlled in 50% of patients with this pattern, akinetic seizures in 37.5%, myoclonic seizures in 35%, and tonic–clonic seizures in two-thirds of patients.

## FELBAMATE

Felbamate was recommended for approval by the Food and Drug Administration in the USA in December 1992 and released for marketing in October 1993. It is currently indicated for use as monotherapy and adjunctive therapy in the treatment of partial seizures with and without generalization in adults with epilepsy, and as adjunctive therapy in the treatment of partial and generalized seizures associated with the Lennox–Gastaut syndrome in children (Pellock, 1994a). The specific approval in children was primarily based on a study wherein 73 patients with Lennox–Gastaut syndrome participated in a multicentre trial that compared the efficacy of felbamate with placebo when administered with background anticonvulsants (Felbamate Study Group in Lennox–Gastaut Syndrome, 1993). This study employed two phases, the first being a 28-day baseline period followed by a 70-day double-blind treatment phase. Patients were monitored in a video telemetry unit to classify seizure type and to determine seizure frequency during a two-day inpatient period which initiated the baseline phase. Parents and guardians were also instructed in the identification of seizure types during the initial hospital admission. During the remainder of the 26-day baseline phase, daily seizure diaries were obtained and patients were treated with fixed doses of standard medications for 26 days as outpatients. At the end of the baseline phase, closed circuit video electroencephalography (EEG) was performed and seizure counts were again recorded. The parent or guardian at that time made a global evaluation of the patient's condition.

The 70-day double-blind treatment phase consisted of a 14-day titration and a 56-day maintenance period. Patients randomized to the felbamate treatment arm of the study received an initial dosage of 15 mg/kg per day, which was increased at weekly intervals to 30 mg/kg per day and then to 45 mg/kg per day or 3600 mg per day, whichever was less, given in four divided doses.

The trial demonstrated that felbamate is effective in the treatment of Lennox–Gastaut syndrome in that it reduced the frequency of atonic, generalized tonic–clonic and total seizures during the study (Figure 2). In addition, according to the parental observation, felbamate improved the overall quality of life by increasing alertness and verbal responsiveness.

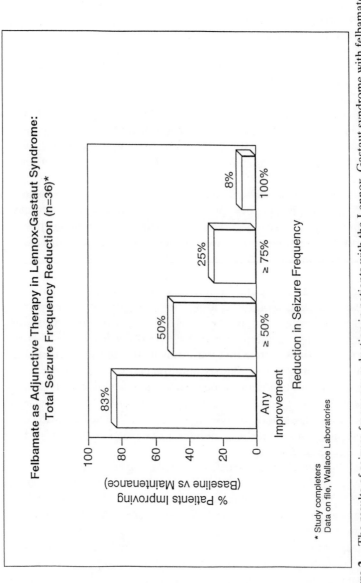
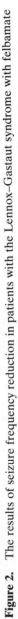

**Figure 2.** The results of seizure frequency reduction in patients with the Lennox–Gastaut syndrome with felbamate

For the purposes of this study, two primary efficacy variables were analysed: (1) comparison between felbamate and placebo treatment groups and
the percentage reduction from baseline in all seizures counted during the
telemetry sessions, and (2) the change in atonic seizure frequency and the
global evaluation as reported by parent or guardian. The global evaluations
encompassed alertness, verbal responsiveness and well-being, and each was
evaluated on a seven-point scale. Efficacy variables were evaluated over the
entire 70-day course of the treatment phase as well as for the 56-day maintenance period of the treatment phase, when the patients were receiving the
maximum study drug doses.

The patients receiving felbamate experienced a mean reduction in
telemetry-monitored seizure frequency of 11%, while the placebo patients
experienced a mean increase of 1%, when the entire treatment phase was
compared with baseline. Although not statistically significant, three patients
treated with felbamate had no seizures during the treatment section, and six
had no seizures during the maintenance period sessions.

Concerning atonic seizures, which were present in 28 patients treated with
felbamate and 22 placebo patients, mean reductions of 34% versus 9% were
reported during the overall treatment phase ($P = 0.01$) while 44% reduction
compared with 7% ($P = 0.002$) was noted during maintenance ($P = 0.002$).
Three patients receiving felbamate had no atonic seizures during the treatment phase, and five had none noted during the maintenance period. Global
evaluation ratings during the maintenance period in the felbamate-treated
group were significantly improved ($P < 0.001$) (Figure 3). Parental counts for
total seizures revealed a 19% reduction for the felbamate-treated group
versus 4% increase in the placebo group ($P = 0.002$) overall. Comparing the
maintenance period to baseline, there was a 26% reduction for patients with
felbamate versus a 5% increase among placebo patients ($P < 0.001$). Four
patients in the felbamate group became seizure-free during the maintenance
period. For generalized tonic–clonic seizures during the maintenance period,
a 40% reduction was noted for the patients on felbamate while a 12% increase was noted in those receiving placebo ($P = 0.017$). Seven patients
treated with felbamate experienced no generalized tonic–clonic seizures during the maintenance period.

Supplemental seizure frequency analyses performed by the manufacturer
(Wallace) revealed that 50% of the 36 felbamate patients completing the trial
had at least a 50% improvement in the frequency of all types of seizures; 69%
had at least a 50% improvement in tonic–clonic seizures; 57% had at least a
50% improvement in atonic seizures; 53% had at least a 50% improvement in
atypical absence seizures; and 50% had at least a 50% improvement in tonic
seizures (Pellock, 1994a). In addition to this initial report, a report of the 12-
month follow-on experience after randomization revealed that the improvement that occurred in the double-blind study was sustained for at least 12

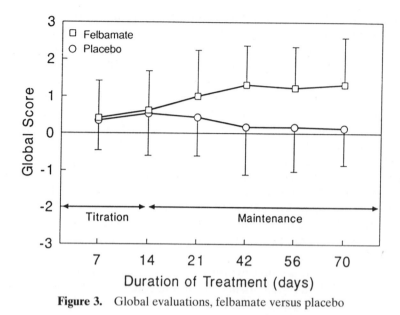

**Figure 3.**    Global evaluations, felbamate versus placebo

months in the subsequent open-label follow-on study (Dodson, 1993b). In the first months of felbamate treatment, 62% of subjects who had previously taken placebo had a reduction in total seizure frequency greater than 50%. By the 12-month follow-up point, approximately half of the patients had a 50% reduction in total seizure count. Atonic seizures responded even better, with two-thirds of patients having a reduction of more than 50% after 12 months' treatment.

The most common adverse reactions seen in association with felbamate administration to children during adjunctive therapy are anorexia, vomiting, insomnia, headache and somnolence. (Pellock, 1994a; Dodson, 1993b; Felbamate Study Group in Lennox–Gastaut Syndrome, 1993). As with all anticonvulsant drugs, most of these symptoms decrease when medication is more slowly initiated and when felbamate is given alone rather than as adjunctive therapy. In two controlled clinical trials, only anorexia tended to persist when patients changed from adjunctive therapy to monotherapy. However, when data from all studies were combined, the incidence of anorexia during monotherapy was approximately one-half that seen during adjunctive therapy. In the Lennox–Gastaut follow-on study, the incidence of anorexia, somnolence and insomnia decreased from 6% for each to 3% for anorexia and somnolence and 1% for insomnia, when comparing the adjunctive and monotherapy groups (Table 1). Overall, in children, the incidence of somnolence in the two groups was 35% versus 11%, anorexia 37% versus 14%, vomiting 25% versus 11%, and insomnia 24% versus 14%, all lower when felbamate

**Table 1.**  Felbamate-related adverse events in children (data to August 1992)

|  | Adjunctive ($n = 306$) | | Monotherapy ($n = 76$) | |
| --- | --- | --- | --- | --- |
|  | n | % | n | % |
| Anorexia | 18 | 6 | 2 | 3 |
| Somnolence | 18 | 6 | 2 | 3 |
| Insomnia | 17 | 6 | 1 | 1 |
| Vomiting | 8 | 3 | 0 | 9 |
| Weight decrease | 5 | 2 | 2 | 3 |
| Nausea | 5 | 2 | 0 | 0 |
| Gait abnormality | 5 | 2 | 0 | 0 |

From Dodson (1993b).

was given alone. In children, only somnolence and anorexia (both 5.8%) and insomnia (5.5%) were considered probably or definitely related to felbamate in various studies, and occurred in more than 5% of patients. No adverse experiences considered severe occurred in children on felbamate alone or as adjuvant therapy.

Because of drug interactions, dosing alterations should be made dependent on adjunctive therapy, and whenever possible felbamate should be given alone (Pellock, 1994a). A titration schedule in which felbamate dosage is increased while other drugs are decreased is suggested. Initial doses of 15 mg/kg per day are recommended, increasing to a maximum of 45 mg/kg per day or 3600 mg. These recommendations for upper dosage limits are based on prior studies. Current usage and ongoing studies suggest that doses of up to 60 mg/kg per day or 4800 mg may yield superior seizure control and are relatively well tolerated (Bebin et al., 1993).

Felbamate appears to be a promising drug for use in children, especially in those with refractory partial and generalized epilepsy. Its role as first-line therapy will need to be further assessed by clinical usage and investigations. Early indications from current trials of the drug in infantile spasms and juvenile myoclonic epilepsy suggest appreciable efficacy.

## GABAPENTIN

Gabapentin has been shown to be efficacious for the treatment of partial seizures in adults (US Gabapentin Study Group No. 5, 1993). The compound was designed to be an analogue of gamma-aminobutyric acid (GABA) with the intention that it would have activity against both generalized and partial seizures. Efficacy and safety trials in children are limited, but are now in progress.

Two studies of identical design were conducted to evaluate the efficacy and safety of gabapentin when used as the initial treatment in children with newly diagnosed absence epilepsy (Leiderman et al., 1993). In the double-blind phase, there was no statistically significant decrease in EEG seizure frequency between the placebo and gabapentin groups. During the open-label phase, which included 21 children, there was a median decrease in percentage change and seizure frequency of 27%, but few children were true responders to gabapentin therapy. With doses of 15–30 mg/kg per day, mild side-effects included somnolence, dizziness, fatigue and headache. It was concluded that gabapentin was no more effective than placebo in suppressing childhood absence seizures, but that therapy for up to 21 months was safe and well tolerated, although ineffective.

A single-centre study was designed to investigate the efficacy and safety of gabapentin in juvenile patients with medically refractory partial seizures. The double-blind, placebo-controlled trial was completed by 8 patients, who then continued into a long-term phase (Parke-Davis data on file). The gabapentin dosing regimen was 20 mg/kg per day, given in three divided doses. Because of the small number of patients, no conclusions could be drawn from the efficacy data.

Most frequently reported adverse effects were convulsions, fever, diarrhoea and conjunctivitis. All patients reported some adverse events. Four patients had clinically important adverse events during the study, which led to withdrawal of three patients.

A double-blind, parallel group comparison of gabapentin versus placebo as add-on therapy for refractory partial epilepsy in children is at present under way in the UK. A trial in benign partial epilepsy in children has been initiated in the USA using gabapentin 20–40 mg/kg versus an active control. Results of these studies will certainly establish whether gabapentin will serve as a useful medication for partial seizures in children. From the results of adult studies, this would be expected.

## LAMOTRIGINE

Lamotrigine is an anticonvulsant drug which is chemically unrelated to currently marketed compounds. It has a preclinical profile suggesting activity against both partial and generalized seizures (Goa et al., 1993). Controlled trials are in progress to determine its efficacy and adverse effect profile in children; however, results are not yet available.

Six open-label, add-on studies were conducted in which 285 of 320 patients with refractory partial and generalized seizures were less than 12 years old (Pellock, 1994b; Wellcome Laboratories, data on file). Following 12 weeks of treatment with lamotrigine, a 26% reduction in seizure frequency was noted in 48% of these children, and a 50% or greater reduction in seizure frequency was noted in 31% of these patients. The initial studies recommended a slow escalation of dosage, from 2 mg/kg initially in induced patients (carbamazepine, phenobarbitone, phenytoin), 1 mg/kg in balanced patients (induced or valproate) and 0.5 mg/kg in patients taking valproate, which inhibits the metabolism of lamotrigine. Subsequent data led to these recommended levels being changed to 2 mg/kg in the first two weeks for induced patients followed by 5 mg/kg in the third and fourth week, with 10 mg/kg recommended thereafter. A maximum of 15 mg/kg or 400 mg is suggested in this group. Patients on valproate with or without other anticonvulsant drugs are recommended to be given 0.5 mg/kg, advanced to 1 mg/kg after the initial two weeks. After four weeks of therapy, the dose is increased to 2 mg/kg with a maximum dose of 5 mg/kg or 200 mg. Using this dosage schedule, efficacy as noted above was similar to that seen in adults with partial seizures. Whether the dose schedules or maximum dose recommendations will be permanent depends upon long-term treatment follow-up in both polypharmacy and monopharmacy lamotrigine studies.

Particularly encouraging is that children with significant neurologic impairment and encephalopathic epilepsy seem to respond as well as the entire pool of children treated with lamotrigine (Hosking *et al.*, 1993). Table 2 compares the percentage of patients with various seizure types achieving a 50% or greater reduction in seizure frequency in severely impaired children versus the total paediatric population treated with lamotrigine. Patients with generalized seizures showed particular benefit, with 53% of patients with typical absence and 50% with atypical absence showing a seizure reduction of 50% or more in the first 12 weeks of lamotrigine treatment. The percentage of patients with a 50% or greater seizure reduction in the first 12 weeks of lamotrigine treatment with myoclonic, clonic, primary generalized and atonic seizures were 31%, 24%, 30% and 38%, respectively. Table 3 compares the efficacy of lamotrigine in various types of seizures in children and adults (Hosking and Spencer, 1993). Studies examining the effects of lamotrigine in children with infantile spasms are under way. A pilot study of monotherapy with lamotrigine in 17 patients with juvenile myoclonic epilepsy is greatly encouraging, suggesting an efficacy equal to valproate (Hosking and Spencer, 1993).

**Table 2.**  Seizure reduction in severely impaired patients treated with lamotrigine

| Patient population | *n* | Patients with reduction of 50% or greater in seizure frequency (%) |
| --- | --- | --- |
| Possible Lennox–Gastaut syndrome | 29 | 37 |
| Severe intellectual impairment | 118 | 36 |
| Paediatric pooled population | 285 | 34 |

From Spencer *et al.*, (1993).

**Table 3.**  Percentage of patients with 50% or greater seizure reduction in first 12 weeks of lamotrigine therapy

| Seizure type | Paediatric $n = 285$ (%) | Adult $n = 677$ (%) |
|---|---|---|
| All | 34 | 32 |
| All partial | 31 | 30 |
| Simple partial | 14 | 24 |
| Complex partial | 34 | 31 |
| Secondary generalized | 33 | 42 |
| Typical absence | 53 | 34 |
| Atypical absence | 50 | 61 |
| Myoclonic | 31 | 31 |
| Clonic | 24 | 36 |
| Primary generalized | 30 | 38 |
| Atonic | 38 | 60 |

From Hosking *et al.*, (1993).

In these patients the adverse effects of lamotrigine include the expected neurotoxicity associated with anticonvulsant drugs. Lamotrigine administration has also been associated with a slightly increased incidence of rash. In children, this drug was well tolerated when added to therapeutic anticonvulsant medications. The most common adverse effects reported by at least 10% of all paediatric patients across all studies were somnolence, skin rash, vomiting, laryngitis and reaction aggravated (increased seizures). At least 5% of these patients reported rhinitis, fever, respiratory disorder, infection, ataxia, hyperkinesia and headache. More serious adverse experiences were reported in 8.8% of these patients, and eight had to stop taking lamotrigine (rash 3, reaction aggravated 3). The most commonly reported adverse experience was reaction aggravated (3.5%) and skin rash (1.1%). The incidence rates for all other serious adverse effects were less than 1%. The percentage of patients discontinuing the drug because of an adverse experience was 12.6%. Skin rash (5.6%), reaction aggravated (1.8%) and somnolence (1.1%) were the most common side-effects leading to discontinuation. Two deaths were reported in children treated with lamotrigine; one was judged to be a sudden unexpected death, the other was judged to be seizure-related (possibly a sudden unexplained death). Neither case was judged to be directly associated with lamotrigine administration. Table 4 compares adverse experiences in paediatric and adult patients (Timmings and Richens, 1993).

Rash associated with lamotrigine therapy needs special consideration. The international experience suggests that withdrawal was not thought necessary when rash occurred in children over six years old, and was not thought to be due to lamotrigine therapy. In cases where lamotrigine was discontinued, the

**Table 4.** Lamotrigine treatment emergent adverse experiences

| Adverse experience | Paediatric n = 285 (%) | Adult n = 677 (%) |
|---|---|---|
| Somnolence | 48 (16.8) | 101 (14.9) |
| All rashes | 47 (16.5) | 43 (6.4) |
| Vomiting | 35 (12.3) | 42 (6.2) |
| Reaction aggravated | 33 (11.6) | 17 (2.5) |
| Fever | 31 (10.9) | 2 (0.3) |

rash was much more common in those receiving concomitant therapy with valproate. The rash rate was examined in relation to the dose of lamotrigine at day 7 in children receiving valproate and lamotrigine. Although the numbers are relatively small, there is a suggestion that within the valproate group the percentage of those developing rash typically received a higher lamotrigine dose. Thus, recommendations for dosing as given above stress very slow escalation of dosing when valproate and lamotrigine are given together.

Although not yet formally tested in children, lamotrigine is reported by patients in long-term studies to result in improved ratings on global scale evaluations (Pellock et al., 1993; Spencer et al., 1993). Some patients anecdotally report a feeling of well-being. This attribute, if it holds true, would be a real benefit in children with epilepsy. The acceptable adverse effect profile and continued efficacy in long-term studies in children and adults suggest that lamotrigine will become a significant part of the anticonvulsant armamentarium both as add-on and monotherapy in children (Hosking et al., 1993).

## OXCARBAZEPINE

Oxcarbazepine is the 10-keto analogue of carbamazepine. Because of its rapid metabolism to an active 10-hydroxy metabolite rather than transformation through carbamazepine 10,11-epoxide, less neurotoxicity is suspected and reported (Grant and Faulds, 1992; Dodson, 1993c). The incidence of rash may also be slightly lower with oxcarbazepine than with carbamazepine. If these findings are confirmed in larger-scale studies in children, the use of oxcarbazepine would certainly be advantageous because of its lower neurologic and systemic toxicity compared with carbamazepine. Although paediatric dosage guidelines are not completely established, a mean daily dose of 1140 mg was reported in one study of 55 children (Klosterskov, 1990).

Oxcarbazepine is indicated primarily for the treatment of partial seizures, and its role in children should be similar. Because of the lack of autoinduction, this drug should be somewhat easier to use than carbamazepine.

## VIGABATRIN

Vigabatrin was the first effective 'tailor-made' anticonvulsant agent and was designed as an irreversible inhibitor of gamma-aminotransferase. As a structural analogue of GABA, it induces a dose-dependent increase in the extracellular content of this inhibitory neurotransmitter. Multiple studies, including those with double-blind, cross-over designs, show it to be efficacious as add-on therapy in adults with refractory partial seizures. Initial studies in children were delayed, as were all trials with vigabatrin in the USA, because of the demonstration of vacuolization in white matter in brains of rodents and dogs. As adults with epilepsy continued to show no evidence of structural or neurophysiologic changes which indicated any white matter changes, studies proceeded in children (Grant and Heel, 1991; Mumford and Dulac, 1991).

Preliminary results of a programme that evaluated vigabatrin as add-on therapy in children with refractory epilepsy were very encouraging; there was a 75–100% decrease in seizure frequency in 25% of patients, with 11 of 135 children becoming seizure-free. Side-effects were reported in 21% of these patients, but were generally transient and rated as severe in only 7 patients (Dulac *et al.*, 1991). Children with partial seizures seemed to show similar benefits to those in adults with difficult-to-control partial epilepsy (Appleton, 1993) (Figure 4). A single patient with Landau–Kleffner syndrome responded dramatically to vigabatrin and carbamazepine in terms of seizure control and reappearance of comprehension and expressive language (Appleton *et al.*, 1993).

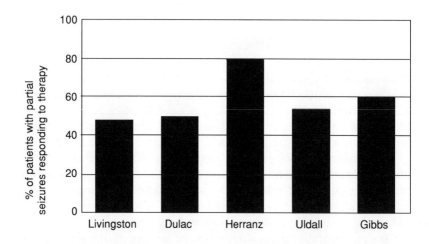

**Figure 4.**   Summary of results from published studies analysing the response of partial seizures to vigabatrin. From Appleton, *Neurol.* 1993; 43(5): S21

In a single-blind, placebo-controlled study, Dulac *et al.* (1991) studied children with severe, intractable epilepsy refractory to all previous drug therapy. Patients were classified as having symptomatic partial, cryptogenic partial, symptomatic generalized, Lennox–Gastaut or non-progressive myoclonic epilepsy. Of 66 patients who entered the active treatment phase of the study, five discontinued the study early because of adverse effects, and three were withdrawn prior to study completion because of worsening of seizures. Of the 58 remaining patients, 29 showed a better than 50% reduction of seizures, and 39 showed a global clinical improvement in their seizure severity. Patients with cryptogenic partial seizures showed the best response, along with patients with Lennox–Gastaut syndrome. Non-progressive myoclonic epilepsy showed the greatest tendency to an increase in seizure frequency, with two of eight children with myoclonic seizures reporting a greater than 50% increase in frequency. Figures 5 and 6 graphically demonstrate the efficacy of vigabatrin according to epilepsy syndrome and seizure type. A clear dose–response relationship could not be ascertained in this small clinical trial, as doses ranged from 25 mg/kg to 125 mg/kg per day. Most patients showing a 90–100% decrease in seizure frequency at the last visit of the trial were receiving doses of 40–80 mg/kg per day. Thus, the recommended starting doses in children following this study were thought to be 40 mg/kg per day increasing to 85 mg/kg per day as necessary (Dulac *et al.*, 1991; Appleton,

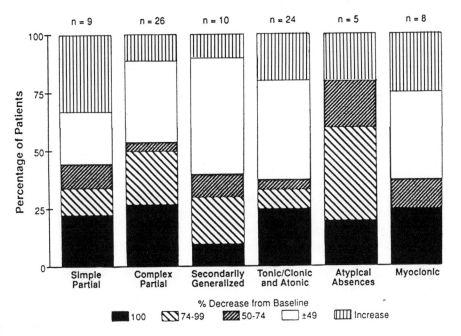

**Figure 5.**   Showing the response of various seizures types to vigabatrin

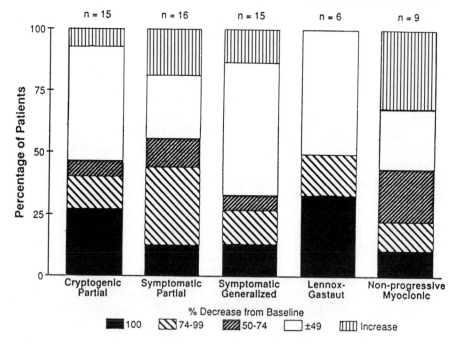

**Figure 6.**   Showing the response of various epilepsy syndromes to vigabatrin

1993). Adverse reactions attributed to vigabatrin during this study included somnolence, stupor, ataxia, hyperkinesia, insomnia, sleep disorder, weight increase and facial oedema. Hyperkinesia was seen in 17 patients (25.7%) and was the most frequently reported adverse event. All of these patients were reported to have some degree of mental retardation or psychiatric problems prior to entering the study, and four exhibited hyperkinesia. Several other authors have reported similar results, with particular success with vigabatrin add-on therapy in children with refractory cryptogenic partial seizures (Appleton, 1993). Even subjects with recurrences after being initially seizure-free seem to have a much lower frequency than recorded at the start of vigabatrin therapy.

Of particular interest is the therapeutic value of vigabatrin in the treatment of refractory infantile spasms. Chiron and colleagues (Chiron *et al.*, 1991) studied 70 children, aged two months to 13 years, who had drug-resistant infantile spasms during the first year of life; of these, 47 were infants. In this open study, in which vigabatrin was given as add-on therapy to the usual anticonvulsant treatment, two children withdrew because of intolerance to vigabatrin, 29 (43%) showed complete suppression of spasms, and 46 children had a greater than 50% reduction in spasms. The best response was observed in those with tuberous sclerosis (12 of 14) compared with those of symptomatic infantile spasms or cryptogenic infantile spasms (Figure 7). Following

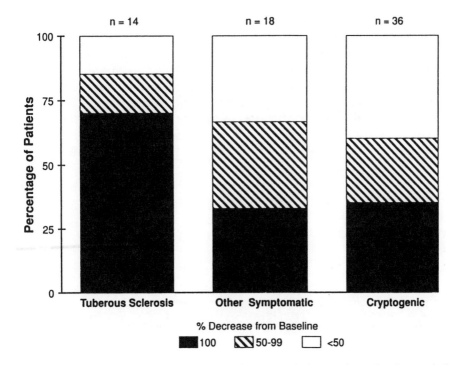

**Figure 7.** Decrease in frequency of infantile spasms during study evaluation period (*n* = 68). From Chiron C *et al., J. Child Neurol.* 1991; 6: S54

the initial response, a long-term response was confirmed in 75% of children with symptomatic infantile spasms and 36% of the children with cryptogenic spasms. In eight children, all other anticonvulsant medications could definitely be withdrawn. Subsequent to this report, some children maintained on vigabatrin alone developed partial seizures and needed the addition of agents such as carbamazepine for full control of their seizures.

Studies of the efficacy of vigabatrin in Lennox–Gastaut syndrome have reported mixed results. The findings of an initial open study of 20 patients were that 60% of children experienced a 60–100% reduction in seizures (Dulac *et al.*, 1991; Mumford and Dulac, 1991; Appleton *et al.*, 1993). Appleton, however, reported disappointing results (Appleton, 1993).

## CONCLUSION

Studies of the newer anticonvulsant drugs suggest exciting additions with improved efficacy and perhaps decreased toxicity in certain types of refractory childhood epilepsy. In some very rare syndromes only anecdotal reports exist and these must be reinforced. Issues of tolerability, long-term safety in very young children, and effects on learning, behaviour and other cognitive functions must be balanced with the possibility of improved efficacy. Continued well-controlled studies in neonates, infants, school-age children and adolescents are much needed, taking into account both seizure types and epilepsy syndromes. A summary of the probable spectrum of new anticonvulsant drugs in childhood seizures and syndromes is given in Table 5.

**Table 5.**   Probable spectrum of new anticonvulsant drugs in childhood epilepsy

| Drug | Seizure/epilepsy type | | | | | |
|---|---|---|---|---|---|---|
| | Partial | Primary generalized | IS | LGS | Myo-clonic | Absence |
| Felbamate | + | + | + | + | + | + |
| Gabapentin | + | +/– | – | – | – | – |
| Lamotrigine | + | + | ? | + | + | + |
| Oxcarbazepine | + | – | – | – | – | – |
| Vigabatrin | + | +/– | + | +/– | – | – |

IS, infantile spasms; LGS, Lennox–Gastaut syndrome; +, efficacious, reported or highly suspected; –, no efficacy proved; +/–, mixed results among population; ?, needs further evaluation, unknown.

## REFERENCES

Appleton RE (1993) The role of vigabatrin in the management of infantile epileptic syndromes. *Neurology,* **43** (5), S21–S23.

Appleton RE, Hughes AP, Beirne M *et al.* (1993) Vigabatrin in the Landau–Kleffner Syndrome. *Dev. Med. Child. Neurol.,* **35,** 457–459.

Bebin EM, Santilli N, Bright S and Dreifuss FE (1993) Results of felbamate dosing for pediatric patients with Lennox–Gastaut Syndrome. *Epilepsia,* **34** (6), 97.

Brantner S and Feucht M (1992) Gamma-vinyl GABA (vigabatrin) in Lennox–Gastaut Syndrome — an open trial (abstract). *Seizure,* **1** (A), 7/05.

Chiron C, Dulac O, Beaumont D *et al.* (1991) Therapeutic trial of vigabatrin in refractory infantile spasms. *J. Child. Neurol.,* **6** (2), 2S52–2S56.

Commission on Antiepileptic Drugs of the International League Against Epilepsy (1991) Workshop on antiepileptic drug trials in children. *Epilepsia,* **32,** 284–285.

Dodson WE (1993a) Pharmacokinetic principles of antiepileptic therapy in children. In: *Pediatric Epilepsy: Diagnosis and Therapy* (eds WE Dodson and JM Pellock), pp 231–240. Demos, New York.

Dodson WE (1993b) Felbamate in the treatment of Lennox–Gastaut Syndrome: results of a 12-month, open-label study following a randomized clinical trial. *Epilepsia,* **34** (7), S18–24.

Dodson WE (1993c) Carbamazepine and oxycarbazepine. In: *Pediatric Epilepsy: Diagnosis and Therapy* (eds WE Dodson and JM Pellock), pp. 303–314. Demos, New York.

Dodson WE and Pellock JM (eds) (1993) *Pediatric Epilepsy: Diagnosis and Therapy.* Demos, New York.

Dulac O, Chiron C, Luna D *et al.* (1991) Vigabatrin in childhood epilepsy. *J. Child. Neurol.,* **6** (2), 2S30–2S37.

Farrell K (1986) Benzodiazepines in the treatment of children with epilepsy. *Epilepsia,* **27** (suppl. 1), 45–51.

Felbamate Study Group in Lennox–Gastaut Syndrome (1993) Efficacy of felbamate in childhood epileptic encephalopathy (Lennox–Gastaut syndrome). *N. Eng. J. Med.,* **328**, 29–33.

Goa KL, Ross SR and Chrisp P (1993) Lamotrigine: a review of its pharmacological properties and clinical efficacy in epilepsy. *Drugs,* **46** (1), 152–176.

Grant SM and Faulds D (1992) Oxcarbazepine: a review of its pharmacology and therapeutic potential in epilepsy, trigeminal neuralgia and affective disorders. *Drugs,* **43** (6), 873–888.

Grant SM and Heel RC (1991) Vigabatrin: a review of its pharmacodynamic and pharmacokinetic properties, and therapeutic potential in epilepsy and disorders of motor control. *Drugs,* **41** (6), 889–926.

Heller AJ, Stewart J, Hughes E and Chesterman P (1993) Comparative efficacy and toxicity of phenobarbital, phenytoin, carbamazepine, and valproate in adults and children with newly diagnosed previously untreated epilepsy: a randomized long-term trial. *Epilepsia,* **34** (2), 66.

Hosking G and Spencer SC (1993) Lamotrigine as add-on therapy in pediatric patients with treatment-resistant epilepsy: an overview. *Epilepsia,* **34** (2), 66.

Hosking G, Spencer S and Yuen AWC (1993) Lamotrigine in children with severe developmental abnormalities in a paediatric population with refractory seizures. *Epilepsia,* **34** (6), 42.

Klosterskov JP (1990) Oxcarbazepine (Trileptal) in anti-epileptic polytherapy. *Behav. Neurol.,* **3** (1), 35–39.

Leiderman D, Garofalo E and LaMoreaux L (1993) Gabapentin patients with absence seizures: two double-blind, placebo controlled studies. *Epilepsia,* **34** (6), 45.

Mumford J and Dulac O (1991) Vigabatrin: a new antiepileptic medication. *J. Child. Neurol.,* **6** (2), 2S3–2S6.

Pellock JM (1989) Efficacy and adverse effects of antiepileptic drugs. *Ped. Clin. N. Amer.,* **36** (2), 435–448.

Pellock JM (1993) Seizures and epilepsy in infancy and childhood. *Neurol. Clin.,* **3** (4), 755–775.

Pellock JM (1994a) Felbamate: the US experience of a new anticonvulsant. *Seizure* (in press).

Pellock JM (1994b) The clinical efficacy of lamotrigine as an antiepileptic drug. *Neurology* (in press).

Pellock JM, Rao C and Earl N (1993) Lamotrigine efficacy and safety update: US experience. *Epilepsia,* **34** (6), 42.

Roger J, Dravet C, Bureau M, Dreifuss FE and Wolf P (1992) *Epileptic Syndromes in Infancy, Childhood and Adolescence.* John Libbey, London.

Spencer SC, Hosking G and Yuen AWC (1993) Experience with long-term lamotrigine treatment as add-on therapy in paediatric patients with treatment-resistant epilepsy. *Epilepsia,* **34** (6), 106.

Timmings PL and Richens A (1993) Efficacy of lamotrigine as monotherapy for juvenile myoclonic epilepsy: pilot study results. *Epilepsia,* **34** (2), 160.

US Gabapentin Study Group No. 5 (1993) Gabapentin as add-on therapy in refractory partial epilepsy: double-blind, placebo-controlled, parallel-group study. *Neurology,* **43**, 2292–2298.

# 10

# Recipes for clinical practice

EMILIO PERUCCA
*University of Pavia, Italy*

## INTRODUCTION

Until 1950, physicians faced few dilemmas when prescribing a drug for the treatment of epilepsy, with only two major agents (phenobarbitone and phenytoin) being available at the time. The next two decades saw the advent of all other 'conventional' anticonvulsants, including primidone (1952), ethosuximide (1958), carbamazepine (1963), benzodiazepines (1965) and sodium valproate (1967). Although the availability of these agents led to major therapeutic advances, rational drug selection became more complicated, and new problems arose with the realization that clinically significant interactions may occur when two or more drugs are prescribed in combination.

After a hiatus of more than 20 years, new anticonvulsant agents have been developed, and many of these have reached the registration stage (Pisani *et al.*, 1991; Perucca, 1993). This implies that the physician treating epilepsy in the late 1990s will be confronted with a therapeutic armamentarium of 15 to 20 drugs. Under these conditions, rational prescribing may become increasingly difficult, especially because no single drug has clearly emerged as outstanding in all seizure types. Some confusion is also likely to develop as a result of conflicting claims rising out of marketing pressure.

The purpose of this chapter is to provide an overview about the role of recently registered drugs in the current management of patients with epilepsy. Although an attempt has been made to justify most considerations on the basis of objective data, comparative drug evaluation is inevitably open to subjective interpretation, and some recommendations may need to be revised as new information becomes available.

*New Anticonvulsants: Advances in the Treatment of Epilepsy.* Edited by M. R. Trimble
© 1994 John Wiley & Sons Ltd

## NEW DRUGS FOR WHICH PATIENTS?

The old anticonvulsant drugs are remarkably effective (Richens and Perucca, 1993). When used appropriately, they produce complete seizure control in approximately two-thirds of treated patients, although the response rate varies in relation to seizure type from excellent (for example, in typical absence seizures) to intermediate (symptomatic partial seizures) or poor (atonic seizures associated with the Lennox–Gastaut syndrome). Patients with 'refractory epilepsy' represent the most obvious candidates for prescription of a new drug.

The need for new drugs, however, is not restricted to these patients. In fact, 'conventional' anticonvulsants exhibit several problems apart from limited efficacy (Table 1). Any new agent possessing a more favourable therapeutic index (for example, a lower toxicity or a reduced interaction potential) could easily be proposed as first-line treatment in newly diagnosed patients. As clearly documented in the preceding chapters of this book, the 'wonder drug' possessing all the desirable properties summarized in Table 2 has yet to be discovered, but some of the new agents do appear to have significant advantages in terms of simple pharmacokinetics, less interference with cognitive functions and lower interaction potential.

**Table 1.**   Some clinical problems associated with old anticonvulsant drugs

Incomplete efficacy

Unfavourable kinetics

Narrow therapeutic ratio

Adverse central nervous system effects

Significant potential for idiosyncratic reactions

Interactions resulting from enzyme induction (carbamazepine, phenytoin, phenobarbitone, primidone) or enzyme inhibition (valproic acid)

**Table 2.**   Ideal properties of an anticonvulsant drug

Known and specific mode of action
Simple kinetics compatible with once or twice daily dosing
No need for complex individualization of dosage
Broad spectrum (efficacy against all seizure types)
Greater efficacy than older drugs
Excellent tolerability — no teratogenic effects
No tolerance or withdrawal effects
No need for plasma level monitoring
No drug interactions — no enzyme induction or inhibition
Availability of a parenteral formulation
Low cost

Since clinical trials of new anticonvulsants almost invariably involve the addition of the test compound to pre-existing therapy in refractory patients, information about the use of new agents as monotherapy is still insufficient to define their potential role as first-line agents in specific seizure types. Based on currently available evidence, therefore, these compounds should be prescribed only in patients who failed to respond to the older drugs (Richens and Perucca, 1993). As discussed below, possible exceptions concern the use of oxcarbazepine in newly diagnosed patients with partial seizures, and the first-line use of vigabatrin in infants with West Syndrome.

## EFFICACY VERSUS SAFETY CONSIDERATIONS

Theoretically, selection of appropriate treatment in the individual patient should be based on knowledge of the comparative efficacy and safety of the various drugs in relation to syndromic form, seizure type and other relevant clinical features (Richens and Perucca, 1993). In practice, however, this information is seldom fully available and much prescribing is based more on subjective perceptions than on sound scientific evidence of superiority of one treatment over another.

This situation is most clearly illustrated by current knowledge about the relative value of the older drugs in different seizure types. Despite the fact that these drugs have been around for more than 20 years and they are usually prescribed as monotherapy, their differential efficacy in relation to type of epilepsy is still incompletely defined. Although few doctors would argue against the preferential use of sodium valproate in the treatment of absence seizures, there is still no consensus about which drug should be prescribed initially in patients with partial or primarily generalized tonic–clonic seizures, the most common seizure types in adults. Indeed, several comparative prospective studies found no differences in efficacy between phenytoin, carbamazepine or valproate in newly diagnosed patients with partial or tonic–clonic seizures (Callaghan *et al.*, 1985; Turnbull *et al.*, 1985; Mattson *et al.*, 1985; Heller *et al.*, 1993). These data led Chadwick and Turnbull (1985) to conclude that no individual drug can be proposed preferentially against these seizure types in adult patients.

To some extent, the inability to detect significant differences in efficacy or tolerability in these studies derives from the low statistical power of many trials. For example, evidence that valproate may in fact be slightly less effective than carbamazepine in the management of complex partial seizures has been provided recently in a multicentre trial which enrolled as many as 480 previously untreated patients (Mattson *et al.*, 1992) but even this finding remains controversial because other large trials failed to detect such a difference (Heller *et al.*, 1993).

With this background, it is no surprise that the comparative efficacy and safety of the newer drugs is very poorly defined, and many years will elapse before reliable information will become available. With a few exceptions, formal comparisons between new drugs and older agents have not been performed, and interpretation of data from separate studies is made difficult by differences in trial design and patient populations. In addition, overall clinical experience with the new drugs is still too limited (especially in patients potentially at special risk, such as infants, the elderly and pregnant women) to allow detection of rare but potentially serious adverse effects. These considerations reinforce the argument that, until further information becomes available, prescription of a new drug should be reserved (with a few exceptions) to patients who failed to respond optimally to conventional treatment. This view is also supported by cost considerations, since the new agents are considerably more expensive than older treatments (Table 3).

Some significant favourable and unfavourable features of new anticonvulsant drugs are summarized in Table 4. The section below discusses the potential role of these agents in the clinical management of patients with specific seizure types.

**Table 3.** Comparative cost of old and new anticonvulsant drugs. Cost is calculated for one-month treatment with lowest cost, non-extended release solid proprietary formulations at the daily dosages indicated. Estimates are based on official 1993 National Health Service prices* in the UK, except for felbamate, oxcarbazepine and zonisamide (unavailable in Britain), whose costs are based on 1993 retail prices in the USA, Denmark and Japan respectively

| Drug | Daily dosages used for estimation (mg/day) | Monthly cost (£ sterling) |
| --- | --- | --- |
| Carbamazepine | 600–1800 | 5.2–15.8 |
| Clonazepam | 4–8 | 5.5–11.0 |
| Ethosuximide | 750–1500 | 6.9–13.8 |
| Phenobarbitone | 60–180 | 0.15–0.45 |
| Phenytoin | 250–400 | 2.1–3.3 |
| Primidone | 500–1500 | 1.1–3.3 |
| Valproic acid | 500–3000 | 3.9–23.7 |
| Clobazam | 20–60 | 7.9–23.8 |
| Felbamate | 2400–3600 | 61.1–91.6 |
| Gabapentin | 900–1800 | 47.7–87.0 |
| Lamotrigine | 100–400 | 30.2–120.7 |
| Oxcarbazepine | 900–2100 | 26.7–57.7 |
| Vigabatrin | 1500–4000 | 41.4–110.4 |
| Zonisamide | 200–600 | 22.6–67.8 |

*Actual price charged by pharmacies in the UK may be greater due to fees and overheads.

**Table 4.** Favourable and unfavourable characteristics of recently developed anticonvulsant drugs

| Drug | Favourable | Unfavourable |
|---|---|---|
| Clobazam | Broad spectrum of activity<br>Remarkable efficacy in some cases | Efficacy short-lived in some patients |
| Felbamate | Promising efficacy in Lennox–Gastaut syndrome | Gastrointestinal symptoms and insomnia<br>Drug interactions |
| Gabapentin | Good tolerability<br>Simple kinetics (at low to intermediate doses)<br>No interactions | Short half-life<br>Limited efficacy |
| Lamotrigine | Broad spectrum<br>Good efficacy in generalized epilepsies | Allergy<br>Drug interactions |
| Oxcarbazepine | Less allergenic, simpler kinetics and lower interaction potential than carbamazepine | Hyponatraemia<br>Interaction with oral contraceptives |
| Vigabatrin | High efficacy<br>Simple kinetics<br>Low interaction risk<br>No allergy<br>No need for TDM | Narrow spectrum<br>Weight gain<br>Adverse psychiatric effects |
| Zonisamide | Broad spectrum<br>Promising activity in myoclonic syndromes | Adverse central nervous system effects<br>Possible urolithiasis |

## ROLE OF THE NEW ANTICONVULSANT DRUGS IN SPECIFIC SEIZURE TYPES

As shown in Table 5, all the new anticonvulsant drugs have been shown to be effective in the management of partial seizures. To some extent, this reflects the fact that for ethical reasons new drugs are evaluated initially in adult patients with refractory epilepsy, and most of these patients have uncontrolled partial seizures. For some drugs, however, evidence about potential activity (or lack of activity) in other seizure types is gradually becoming available, allowing some preliminary suggestions to be made about rational prescribing.

**Table 5.** Response rate to recently developed anticonvulsant drugs used add-on in patients with (mostly) refractory partial seizures, with or without secondary generalization. Response rate is defined as the percentage of patients who achieved a 50% or greater reduction in seizure frequency (versus placebo) in double-blind, placebo-controlled, short-term trials. When results were originally expressed as changes versus baseline, the placebo response (or the response in the placebo group, for parallel group designs) was subtracted from the response rate during drug treatment. For parallel group designs, number of patients excludes patients treated with placebo

|  | Percentage of patients with 50% or greater response | Number of trials | Number of patients | Reference |
|---|---|---|---|---|
| Felbamate | 16 | 2 | 84 | Anonymous (1993) |
| Gabapentin | 9–15 | 3 | 422 | Brown (1993) |
| Lamotrigine | 22 | 7 | 283 | Brodie (1992) |
| Oxcarbazepine | No placebo-controlled studies available |  |  |  |
| Vigabatrin | 40 | 8 | 258 | Mumford and Dam (1989); Marion–Merrell–Dow, data on file |
| Zonisamide | 21 | 1 | 71 | Schmidt, Jacob, Loiseau *et al.* (1993) |

## Partial seizures (with or without secondary generalization)

A comparison of response rates (versus placebo) observed in randomized double-blind, add-on trials of new anticonvulsant drugs in patients with (mostly) partial seizures resistant to conventional agents is presented in Table 5. These data should be interpreted cautiously because study designs and experimental conditions were highly variable, and response rates tended to show marked intertrial differences even with the same drug. In the case of lamotrigine, for example, the percentage of patients showing a good to excellent response ranged in different trials from 67% to 11% (Richens and Yuen, 1991).

Despite these limitations of interpretation, available data suggest that vigabatrin produces the most favourable results when given as add-on therapy to patients with refractory partial seizures. Therefore, it is reasonable to suggest that vigabatrin should be used preferentially in patients with partial seizures uncontrolled by conventional agents. In the author's opinion, vigabatrin could be proposed as the next agent to be used in patients who failed an initial trial of the first-line drug, which is usually carbamazepine. In fact, vigabatrin may be superior to phenytoin and phenobarbitone in terms of non-interference with cognitive function (McGuire *et al.*, 1992), while valproate may be less effective in the management of partial seizures (Mattson *et al.*, 1992). Further advantages of vigabatrin include a low interaction potential, long-term tolerability (Tartara *et al.*, 1992) and the lack of need for serum drug level monitoring. Vigabatrin should not be used (or should be used with extreme caution) in patients with a history of psychiatric or personality disorders, and in patients with associated myoclonic seizures. One disadvantage of vigabatrin is that it has not been adequately assessed as monotherapy, and therefore it will have to be used as add-on medication. This is in contrast with the commonly recommended practice of substituting monotherapy with a second drug when patients do not respond fully to initial treatment.

If add-on vigabatrin has been ineffective or there are conditions contraindicating its use, it is probably wise to select one of the older agents such as valproate or phenytoin. In patients refractory to conventional drugs, acceptable alternatives are represented by lamotrigine (Richens and Yuen, 1991), gabapentin (UK Gabapentin Study Group, 1990; Foot and Wallace, 1991; Leiderman *et al.*, 1993), zonisamide (Peters and Sorkin, 1993) and felbamate (Leppik *et al.*, 1991; Sachdeo *et al.*, 1992). Selection among these agents is largely dictated by current availability in individual countries, with lamotrigine being more prevalent in Europe and zonisamide being restricted to the Far East. Preliminary uncontrolled observations suggest that lamotrigine may be more effective in patients with generalized epilepsies (Yuen, 1991; Timmings and Richens, 1992), but encouraging results with this drug are reported also in a considerable proportion of patients with partial seizures (Richens and Yuen, 1991), including some receiving lamotrigine as monotherapy (Study 106 Investigators *et al.*, 1993).

With gabapentin, there is preliminary evidence that complex partial seizures and secondarily generalized seizures respond better than simple partial seizures (Leiderman *et al.*, 1993).

Oxcarbazepine occupies an unusual place in this context. This compound is considered to act by the same mechanism as carbamazepine and therefore it would be illogical to prescribe it in patients whose seizures failed to respond to carbamazepine, although scientific proof for this is lacking (Editorial, 1989). Conversely, oxcarbazepine would be a reasonable choice in patients who had to discontinue carbamazepine because of a skin rash.

Oxcarbazepine is the only new drug that has undergone relatively extensive monotherapy evaluation in newly diagnosed patients with partial seizures. In the Scandinavian trial, the proportion of previously untreated patients who achieved complete seizure control on oxcarbazepine was not significantly different from the carbamazepine group (Dam *et al.*, 1989). The incidence of side-effects was comparable with the two drugs, but adverse effects leading to discontinuation of treatment (mostly skin rashes) were twice as common in the carbamazepine group. Although these results suggest that oxcarbazepine may be at least as valuable as carbamazepine in the management of adult patients with partial seizures, interpretation of data is complicated by inadequate description of the study population. For example, patients with primarily generalized tonic–clonic seizures were also included in the study, and no data were provided about the distribution of seizure types in the two groups, or about the response in relation to seizure type.

A review of available evidence suggests that oxcarbazepine is comparable to carbamazepine in anticonvulsant efficacy and offers some advantages in terms of simpler and less variable pharmacokinetics, less allergenic potential, lower enzyme-inducing activity and less susceptibility to drug interactions (Grant and Faulds, 1992). On the other hand, hyponatraemia is much more common during treatment with oxcarbazepine than with carbamazepine, and in a few patients this effect may be troublesome (Steinhoff et al., 1992). Whether the above-mentioned advantages outweigh the hyponatraemic risk (and the drawback of less extensive safety and efficacy data compared with carbamazepine) is a matter of personal judgement. Although individual physicians may consider using oxcarbazepine as the drug of choice in patients with newly diagnosed partial seizures, it is the author's opinion that further studies are required before this drug can be proposed for the first-line therapy in such patients.

### Primary generalized tonic–clonic seizures

Most physicians today consider valproate as the drug of choice for the treatment of primary generalized tonic–clonic seizures. Alternative treatments for patients who failed to respond to valproate include carbamazepine, phenytoin, phenobarbitone, lamotrigine and, possibly, zonisamide. Selection among these drugs will depend on individual factors such as the practitioner's experience with a given agent, the importance of avoiding sedative effects (especially marked with barbiturates), the age of the patient (phenytoin and barbiturates are best avoided in childhood), the desire to avoid interactions with the contraceptive pill (phenytoin, carbamazepine and barbiturates stimulate the metabolism of contraceptive steroids), and cost considerations.

Available information is insufficient to justify an early trial of felbamate or gabapentin, and vigabatrin is usually considered to be less effective in generalized seizures than in the partial epilepsies (Grant and Heel, 1991). On the other hand, lamotrigine has been reported to be particularly valuable in the management of primarily generalized tonic–clonic seizures (Yuen, 1991; Sander et al., 1991; Timmings and Richens, 1992), and it may be reasonable to use it preferentially to the other new drugs in these patients. Zonisamide has also been reported to be effective in this seizure type (Peters and Sorkin, 1993).

## Absence seizures

Valproate is generally regarded as the treatment of choice in absence seizures. Patients whose seizures fail to be controlled by valproate may benefit from ethosuximide or, in the case of atypical absence seizures, a combination of valproate with ethosuximide (Richens and Perucca, 1993). Good results in patients with absence seizures have been reported with both lamotrigine (Sander et al., 1991; Yuen, 1991) and zonisamide (Peters and Sorkin, 1993). A favourable synergistic interaction between valproate and lamotrigine in this seizure type has also been reported (Panayiotopoulos et al., 1993).

Absence seizures usually are not improved and may even be worsened by administration of vigabatrin (Grant and Heel, 1991; Gibbs et al., 1992).

## Atonic seizures and the Lennox–Gastaut syndrome

Information about the efficacy of individual drugs on this seizure type is still insufficient, with the possible exception of felbamate. A double-blind, placebo-controlled trial has demonstrated a dose-dependent favourable effect of felbamate on the frequency of atonic seizures associated with the Lennox–Gastaut syndrome (Felbamate Study Group in Lennox–Gastaut Syndrome, 1993). These seizures are severely disabling and usually refractory to treatment, and therefore a trial of felbamate would be justified in this condition.

Open studies have also suggested a potential usefulness of lamotrigine (Yuen, 1991; Oller et al., 1993) and zonisamide (Peters and Sorkin, 1993) in this seizure type, and lamotrigine has been proposed as the initial treatment of choice for children with the Lennox–Gastaut syndrome (Dulac, 1993). Several authors have reported improved seizure control with add-on vigabatrin in some children with the Lennox–Gastaut syndrome (Dulac et al., 1991; Brantner and Feucht, 1992), although response to vigabatrin is generally regarded as disappointing in this condition (R.E. Appleton, personal communication). Controlled trials with these drugs are awaited in order to assess the significance of these observations.

## Myoclonic seizures

Myoclonic seizures are usually treated with valproate, and it has been suggested that patients unresponsive to valproate alone may benefit from addition of a benzodiazepine (Richens and Perucca, 1993). When this strategy fails, trial of a new agent appears to be justified. Preliminary data suggest that zonisamide may be particularly valuable in the add-on treatment of myoclonic seizures, especially in patients with autosomal recessive Baltic myoclonus epilepsy (Henry et al., 1988), and the drug is available for compassionate use in Scandinavia (E. Ben-Menachem, personal communication).

Lamotrigine has also been reported to be effective in myoclonic seizures (Yuen, 1991), although some patients may not respond favourably to this drug (Sander *et al.*, 1991). A recent study indicated that lamotrigine may also be valuable as monotherapy for the management of juvenile myoclonic epilepsy (Timmings and Richens, 1993).

Vigabatrin is not recommended for patients with this seizure type since it may worsen the condition and even cause myoclonus in some cases (Grant and Heel, 1991; Gibbs *et al.*, 1992; Buti *et al.*, 1993b).

### Infantile spasms (West syndrome)

Vigabatrin has been reported to be remarkably effective in suppressing infantile spasms in a considerable proportion of cases, especially in patients with tuberous sclerosis (Chiron *et al.*, 1991; Gram *et al.*, 1992). There are also preliminary favourable results with the use of this drug as monotherapy (Appleton and Montiel-Viesca, 1992; Buti *et al.*, 1993a). Therefore, there is a justification for the use of this drug in patients unresponsive to steroid or valproate therapy. Effective daily doses are usually in the 40–80 mg/kg range, but doses up to 150 mg/kg have also been used. The response to vigabatrin is usually maintained over time, although some patients (especially those with cryptogenic spasms) may relapse after a few months (Gram *et al.*, 1992).

Since vigabatrin is usually relatively well tolerated, while steroids may produce severe adverse effects and valproate rarely induces liver toxicity, a case has been made for the early use of vigabatrin as first-line therapy in patients with infantile spasms (Appleton and Montiel-Viesca, 1992), at least in the subgroup with the symptomatic type (Dulac, 1993). Response can usually be assessed within a few days, and an alternative treatment can be instituted rapidly should vigabatrin be ineffective.

## USE OF THE NEW ANTICONVULSANT DRUGS IN SPECIAL CONDITIONS

### Infants and children

In general, experience with the new drugs in children is still limited and further clinical trials need to be performed before specific indications and dosage recommendations can be made. Possible exceptions are vigabatrin, for which there is relatively extensive evidence to justify its paediatric use as add-on medication, especially in refractory partial seizures (Gram *et al.*, 1992), lamotrigine (Hosking and Spencer, 1993) and zonisamide (Shuto *et al.*, 1989; Peters and Sorkin, 1993). The latter two drugs may be valuable in the management of a broad range of seizure types in children.

The role of vigabatrin in the management of infantile spasms and the value of felbamate and other drugs in the treatment of the Lennox–Gastaut syndrome has been discussed above.

## Women with childbearing potential

Some of the new anticonvulsant drugs, such as lamotrigine, felbamate and gabapentin, have been found to be devoid of teratogenic effects in animal toxicology testing, and there is hope that these compounds could also be less risky to the human fetus than the old drugs. Unfortunately, animal data are not fully predictive of human teratogenic potential, and prescription of these drugs is usually discouraged in women likely to become pregnant.

Phenobarbitone, carbamazepine, primidone and phenytoin (but not sodium valproate) induce the metabolism of steroid oral contraceptives and reduce the efficacy of the contraceptive pill. Lamotrigine (Holdich et al., 1991) and gabapentin (Busch et al., 1993) offer the advantage of not interfering with the contraceptive pill, and this could be an important consideration when selecting treatment in female patients. Vigabatrin, which is eliminated unchanged in urine without hepatic metabolism, is also expected not to interact with the pill, but this requires formal confirmation. Although oxcarbazepine is generally considered to have a lower enzyme-inducing potency than carbamazepine, it has been shown to stimulate steroid metabolism and to decrease contraceptive efficacy (Grant and Faulds, 1992; Jensen et al., 1992). There is some evidence that felbamate may also act as an enzyme inducer, but its potential interaction with the contraceptive pill has not been investigated.

## The elderly

It is generally recommended that cerebrally active drugs be used with special caution in the elderly, because of the risks related to altered pharmacokinetics and increased central nervous system sensitivity. In particular, kidney function is reduced in old age, resulting in reduced clearance of renally eliminated drugs such as vigabatrin and gabapentin. In the case of vigabatrin, there is evidence that elderly patients may develop toxic effects such as drowsiness and confusion after intake of doses that are well tolerated in the young (Haegele et al., 1988). The elderly also appear to be at greater risk of developing oxcarbazepine-induced symptomatic hyponatraemia (Pendlebury et al., 1989; Steinhoff et al., 1992), and a decrease in the clearance of the active 10-hydroxy-metabolite of oxcarbazepine has been reported in old patients (Grant and Faulds, 1992). The elderly also show a moderate decrease in rate of lamotrigine elimination (Posner et al., 1991).

**Hepatic and renal disease**

Drugs that are eliminated by oxidative biotransformation often show reduced clearance in the presence of severe hepatic disease such as liver cirrhosis, while conjugation is often relatively spared (McLean and Morgan, 1991). Since lamotrigine is metabolized by glucuronide conjugation, its metabolism would not be expected to be greatly affected by liver disease, although this requires adequate evaluation. Drugs eliminated by the renal route (e.g. gabapentin and vigabatrin) show potential advantages when treating patients with liver disease, but caution is always required because the central nervous system sensitivity to drugs is often altered in the presence of hepatic failure (McLean and Morgan, 1991).

Renal insufficiency may result in clinically significant accumulation of renally eliminated drugs or active metabolites. Drugs that are not metabolized, such as vigabatrin and gabapentin, should be used with extreme caution and at appropriately modified dosages in these patients. The elimination of 10-hydroxycarbazepine, the active metabolite of oxcarbazepine, may also be impaired in patients with severe renal failure (S. Schwabe, personal communication).

**Miscellaneous conditions**

A number of pathological conditions may dictate special strategies in drug selection. For example, a history of psychiatric disease may predispose to vigabatrin-induced behavioural or psychotic reactions, and it should be considered as a relative contraindication to the use of this drug (Sander and Hart, 1990). Conversely, vigabatrin appears to be remarkably free of allergenic potential, and it may be reasonable to select it preferentially in patients with a known history of frequent or severe immunologically mediated adverse drug reactions. Since oxcarbazepine has marked antidiuretic effects, it should be used cautiously in patients prone to develop electrolyte disturbances.

Most of the old anticonvulsant drugs can precipitate attacks of acute intermittent porphyria in susceptible patients. Since enzyme induction is often associated with precipitation of porphyric attacks, there is hope that some of the newer drugs devoid of inducing effects might be used safely in these patients. Of course, this possibility requires evaluation.

## DRUG INTERACTIONS BETWEEN OLD AND NEW ANTICONVULSANT DRUGS

Drug interactions between anticonvulsants may be a major problem (Pisani *et al.*, 1990). The availability of new drugs, by increasing the number of possible drug combinations, also increases the number of potentially significant interactions to which patients with epilepsy are exposed (see Chapter 1). On the other hand, many of the new drugs exhibit a lower interaction potential compared with the older agents, and this may result in an overall decrease in the size of the problem.

Vigabatrin and gabapentin stand out prominently for their particularly low risk of interaction (Perucca and Pisani, 1991). Both agents appear to be devoid of enzyme inducing or inhibiting potential, and their kinetics are unaffected by concomitantly taken anticonvulsants.

Lamotrigine does not appear to influence the kinetics of other drugs, but its own metabolism is markedly affected by concurrent medication (Peck, 1991). A favourable synergistic interaction between lamotrigine and valproate has been proposed in patients with absence seizures (Panayiotopoulos et al., 1993) and complex partial seizures (Pisani et al., 1993).

The interaction potentials of felbamate and zonisamide are incompletely defined. Felbamate, however, may increase the serum levels of phenytoin and valproic acid, while zonisamide may increase serum carbamazepine. Although felbamate lowers serum carbamazepine, it increases serum carbamazepine 10,11-epoxide and in some cases it may precipitate signs of carbamazepine intoxication if the carbamazepine dose is not reduced. The metabolism of both felbamate and zonisamide is stimulated by concurrently taken enzyme-inducing anticonvulsants (Perucca and Pisani, 1991).

## DRUG INTERACTIONS BETWEEN NEW ANTICONVULSANT DRUGS

Although combination therapy with two or more of the new anticonvulsants is generally not recommended, it is inevitable that their increasing use will eventually lead to simultaneous prescription. Information about the effect of combining new anticonvulsant drugs is virtually lacking, except for the lamotrigine-vigabatrin combination. Since lamotrigine is considered to reduce excessive excitation while vigabatrin acts by potentiating GABAergic inhibition, it has been suggested that these drugs may exert favourable complementary actions. Preliminary clinical observations do suggest the occurrence of a synergistic pharmacodynamic interaction when these agents are combined (Stewart et al., 1992; Robinson et al., 1993; Stolarek et al., 1993).

## CONCLUSION

Although data on the clinical pharmacology and therapeutic value of the new anticonvulsant drugs are still grossly incomplete, available information does allow some suggestions to be made about rational prescribing in specific situations. These agents have not solved completely the problem of drug-resistant epilepsy, but their availability is welcome in the management of selected patients.

Further studies and wider clinical experience are required to assess in greater detail the risk–benefit ratio and the cost-effectiveness of individual agents before any of these can be proposed for the first-line treatment of specific syndromic forms or seizure types.

## REFERENCES

Anonymous (1993) *Felbamate. A Novel Antiepileptic Agent.* Churchill Radius, Clifton, NJ.

Appleton RE and Montiel-Viesca F (1992) Vigabatrin in infantile spasms — why add-on? *Lancet,* **341**, 962.

Brantner S and Feucht M (1992) Gamma-vinyl-GABA (vigabatrin) in the Lennox Gastaut syndrome. An open trial. *Seizure,* **1** (suppl. A), abstract.

Brodie M (1992) Lamotrigine. *Lancet,* **339**, 1397–1400.

Brown TR (1993) Efficacy and safety of gabapentin. In: *New Trends in Epilepsy Management: The Role of Gabapentin* (ed. D. Chadwick), pp. 47–57. Royal Society of Medicine, London.

Busch JA, Bockbrader H, Randinitis EJ *et al.* (1993) Lack of clinically significant drug interactions with Neurontin (gabapentin). *Epilepsia,* **34** (suppl. 2), 158.

Buti D, Lini M, Rota M *et al.* (1993a) Vigabatrin (GVG) in infantile spasms (IS): results in 14 children. *Epilepsia,* **34** (suppl. 2), 94.

Buti D, Rota M, Marvulli I, Nencioli C, Tromboni P and Lini M (1993b) Myoclonus induced by gamma-vinyl GABA (vigabatrin, GVG) in 3 children with infantile spasms. *Epilepsia,* **34** (suppl. 2), 118–119.

Callaghan N, Kenny RA, O'Neil B, Crowley M and Goggin T (1985) A prospective study between carbamazepine, phenytoin and sodium valproate as monotherapy in previously untreated and recently diagnosed patients with epilepsy. *J. Neurol. Neurosurg. Psychiatry,* **48**, 639–645.

Chadwick D and Turnbull DM (1985) The comparative efficacy of antiepileptic drugs for partial and tonic–clonic seizures. *J. Neurol. Neurosurg. Psychiatry,* **48**, 1073–1080.

Chiron C, Dulac O, Beaumont D, Palacios L, Pajot N and Mumford JP (1991) Therapeutic trial of vigabatrin in refractory infantile spasms. *J. Child Neurol.,* **6** (suppl. 2), 52–59.

Dam M, Ekberg R, Lovning Y, Waltimo O and Jakobsen K (1989) A double-blind study comparing oxcarbazepine and carbamazepine in patients with newly diagnosed, previously untreated epilepsy. *Epilepsy Res.,* **3**, 70–76.

Dulac O (1993) Rational use of antiepileptic drugs in children. *Epilepsia,* **39** (suppl. 2), 188.

Dulac O, Chiron C, Cusmai R, Pajot N, Beaumont D and Mondragon S (1991) Vigabatrin in childhood epilepsy. *J. Child Neurol.,* **6** (suppl.), 2S30–2S37.

Editorial (1989) Oxcarbazepine. *Lancet,* **ii**, 196–197.

Felbamate Study Group in Lennox–Gastaut Syndrome (1993) Efficacy of felbamate in childhood epileptic encephalopathy (Lennox–Gastaut syndrome). *N. Eng. J. Med.,* **328**, 29–33.

Foot M and Wallace J (1991) Gabapentin. In: *New Antiepileptic Drugs* (eds F Pisani, E Perucca, G Avanzini and A Richens), pp. 109–114. Elsevier, Amsterdam.

Gibbs JM, Appleton RE and Rosenbloom L (1992) Vigabatrin in intractable childhood epilepsy: a retrospective study. *Pediat. Neurol.,* **8**, 338–340.

Gram L, Sabers A and Dulac O (1992) Treatment of pediatric epilepsies with gamma-vinyl-GABA (vigabatrin). *Epilepsia*, **33** (suppl. 5), S26–S29.

Grant M and Faulds D (1992) Oxcarbazepine. A review of its pharmacology and therapeutic efficacy in epilepsy, trigeminal neuralgia and affective disorders. *Drugs*, **43**, 837–888.

Grant SM and Heel RC (1991) Vigabatrin. A review of its pharmacodynamic and pharmacokinetic properties, and therapeutic potential in epilepsy and disorders of motor control. *Drugs*, **41**, 889–926.

Haegele K, Huebert ND, Ebel M, Tell G and Schechter PJ (1988) Pharmacokinetics of vigabatrin, Implications of creatinine clearance. *Clin. Pharmacol. Therap.*, **44**, 558–565.

Heller AJ, Stewart J, Hughes E *et al.* (1993) Comparative efficacy and toxicity of phenobarbital, phenytoin, carbamazepine, and valproate in adults and children with newly diagnosed previously untreated epilepsy, a randomized long-term trial. *Epilepsia*, **34** (suppl. 2), 66.

Henry TR, Leppik IE, Gumnit RJ and Jacobs MP (1988) Progressive myoclonus epilepsy treated with zonisamide. *Neurology*, **38**, 928–931.

Holdich T, Whiteman P, Orme M, Back D and Wards S (1991) Effect of lamotrigine on the pharmacology of the combined oral contraceptive pill. *Epilepsia*, **32** (suppl. 1), 96).

Hosking G and Spencer SC (1993) Lamotrigine as add-on therapy in pediatric patients with treatment resistant epilepsy: an overview. *Epilepsia*, **34** (suppl. 2), 66.

Jensen PK, Saano V, Haring P, Svenstrup P and Menge GP (1992) Possible interaction between oxcarbazepine and an oral contraceptive. *Epilepsia*, **33**, 1149–1152.

Leiderman D, Anhut H, Sauermann W and Baron B (1993) Response to gabapentin by type of partial seizure. *Epilepsia*, **34** (suppl. 2), 182.

Leppik IE, Dreifuss FE, Pledger GW *et al.* (1991) Felbamate for partial seizures: results of a controlled clinical trial. *Neurology*, **41**, 1785–1789.

Mattson RH, Cramer JA, Collins JF *et al.* (1985) Comparison of carbamazepine, phenobarbital, phenytoin, and primidone in partial and secondarily generalized tonic–clonic seizures. *N. Engl. J. Med.*, **313**, 145–151.

Mattson RH, Cramer JA, Collins JF and the Department of VA Epilepsy Cooperative Study No 264 Group (1992) A comparison of valproate with carbamazepine for the treatment of complex partial seizures and secondarily generalized tonic–clonic seizures in adults. *N. Eng. J. Med.*, **327**, 765–771.

McLean AJ and Morgan DJ (1991) Clinical pharmacokinetics in patients with liver disease. *Clin. Pharmacokin.*, **21**, 42–69.

McGuire AM, Duncan JS and Trimble MR (1992) Effects of vigabatrin on cognitive function and mood when used as add-on therapy in patients with intractable epilepsy. *Epilepsia*, **33**, 128–134.

Mumford JP and Dam M (1989) Meta-analysis of European placebo-controlled studies of vigabatrin in drug-resistant epilepsy. *Br. J. Clin. Pharmacol.*, **27** (suppl. 1), 101–106S.

Oller LFV and Oller Daurella L (1993) Lamotrigine in the treatment of symptomatic generalized epilepsy, particularly Lennox–Gastaut syndrome. *Epilepsia*, **34** (suppl. 2), 66.

Panayiotopoulos CP, Ferrie CD, Knott C and Robinson RO (1993) Interaction of lamotrigine with sodium valproate. *Lancet*, **341**, 445.

Peck AW (1991) Clinical pharmacology of lamotrigine. *Epilepsia*, **32** (suppl. 2), S9–12.

Pendlebury SC, Moses DK and Eadie MJ (1989) Hyponatriemia during oxcarbazepine therapy. *Hum. Toxicol.*, **8**, 337–344.

Perucca E (1993) The clinical pharmacology of new antiepileptic drugs. *Pharmacol. Res.*, **28**, 89–106.

Perucca E and Pisani F (1991) Pharmacokinetics and interactions of the new antiepileptic drugs. In: *New Antiepileptic Drugs* (eds F Pisani, E Perucca, G Avanzini and A Richens), pp. 79–88. Elsevier, Amsterdam.

Peters DH and Sorkin EM (1993) Zonisamide. A review of its pharmacodynamic and pharmacokinetic properties, and therapeutic potential in epilepsy. *Drugs*, **45**, 760–787.

Pisani F, Perucca E and Di Perri R (1990) Clinically relevant antiepileptic drug interactions. *J. Int. Med. Res.*, **18**, 1–15.

Pisani F, Perucca E, Avanzini G and Richens A, eds (1991) *New Antiepileptic Drugs*. Elsevier, Amsterdam.

Pisani F, Perucca E, Richens A and Di Perri R (1993) Interaction of lamotrigine with sodium valproate. *Lancet*, **341**, 1224.

Posner J, Holdich T and Crome P (1991) Comparison of lamotrigine pharmacokinetics in young and elderly healthy volunteers. *J. Pharm. Med.*, **1**, 121–128.

Richens A and Perucca E (1993) Clinical pharmacology and medical treatment. In: *A Textbook of Epilepsy* (eds J Laidlaw, A Richens and D Chadwick), pp. 495–559. Churchill Livingstone, Edinburgh.

Richens A and Yuen WC (1991) Overview of the clinical efficacy of lamotrigine. *Epilepsia*, **32** (suppl. 2), S13–16.

Robinson MK, Black AB, Schapel GS and Lam E (1993) Combined gamma-vinyl GABA (vigabatrin) and lamotrigine therapy in management of refractory epilepsy. *Epilepsy*, **34** (suppl. 2), 109.

Sachdeo R, Kramer LD, Rosenberg A and Sachdeo S (1992) Felbamate monotherapy. Controlled trial in patients with partial onset seizures. *Ann. Neurol.*, **32**, 386–392.

Sander JWAS and Hart YM (1990) Vigabatrin and behaviour disturbances. *Lancet*, **335**, 57.

Sander JWAS, Hart YM, Patsalos PN, Duncan JS and Shorvon SD (1991) Lamotrigine and generalized seizures. *Epilepsia*, **32** (suppl. 1), 59.

Schmidt D, Jacob R, Loiseau P et al. (1993) Zonisamide for add-on treatment of refractory partial epilepsy: a European double blind trial. *Epilepsy Res.*, **15**, 67–73.

Shuto H, Sugimoto T, Yasuhara A et al. (1989) Efficacy of zonisamide in children with refractory partial seizures. *Curr. Ther. Res.*, **45**, 1031–1036.

Steinhoff BJ, Stoll KD, Stodieck SRG and Paulus W (1992) Hyponatremic coma under oxcarbazepine therapy. *Epilepsy Res.*, **11**, 67–70.

Stewart J, Hughes E and Reynolds EH (1992) Lamotrigine for generalized epilepsies. *Lancet*, **340**, 1223.

Stolarek I, Blacklaw J, Thompson GG and Brodie MJ (1993) Gamma-vinyl GABA (vigabatrin) and lamotrigine, synergism in refractory epilepsy? *Epilepsia*, **34** (suppl. 2), 108–109.

Study 106 Investigators, Yuen AWC and Chapman A (1993) Interim report on an open multicenter lamotrigine (Lamictal) versus carbamazepine monotherapy trial in patients with epilepsy. *Epilepsia*, **34** (suppl. 2), 159.

Tartara A, Manni R, Galimberti CA et al. (1992) Six-year follow-up study on the efficacy and safety of vigabatrin in patients with epilepsy. *J. Neurol. Neurosurg. Psychiatry*, **86**, 247–251.

Timmings PL and Richens A (1992) Lamotrigine in primary generalized epilepsy. *Lancet*, **339**, 1300–1301.

Timmings PL and Richens A (1993) Effect of lamotrigine as monotherapy for juvenile myoclonic epilepsy: pilot study results. *Epilepsia*, **34** (suppl. 2), 160.

Turnbull DM, Howell D, Rawlins MD and Chadwick DW (1985) Which drug for this adult epileptic patient, phenytoin or valproate? *Br. Med. J.,* **290**, 815–820.

UK Gabapentin Study Group (1990) Gabapentin in partial epilepsy. *Lancet,* **335**, 114–117.

Yuen AWC (1991) Lamotrigine. In: *New Antiepileptic Drugs* (eds F Pisani, E Perucca, G Avanzini and A Richens), pp. 115–123. Elsevier, Amsterdam.

# Index

*Index compiled by Jill Halliday*